The Athletic Hunter

Sportsmedicine for the Outdoorsman

by Jeffry Metheny, M.D.

DAVID & SANDY —
    IN & AROUND HODGES CABIN
EVERY SEASON IS AN AEROBIC ONE.
THANKS for OPENING YOUR DOOR,
YOUR HEARTS & A BEER OR 2 —
                                JEFF

Double Gauge Press
Davis, California

ISBN: 0-9634193-0-7

Typesetting, Camera-ready Production and Printing Coordination by:
GRAPHIC GOLD
P.O. Box 1582, Davis, California 95617

Illustrations by Janet Williams

Cover Design by Kathi Zamminer

Manufactured in the United States of America.

Foreword

Growing up with organized, team sports we learn to appreciate discipline, teamwork, sportsmanship, camaraderie, and work ethic. The forest, the stream, and all things wild teach us as well, but on a more subtle and introspective level. From the first day we cross a barbed wire fence, shoot a .22, or drink a cup of coffee before sunrise we are taught respect.

Respect your firearm. Never should it mistakenly harm anything or anyone. Clean it, polish it, and it will become a trusted friend, much like a well worn baseball glove.

Respect the land, handle her gently, her recovery and regenerating potential is immense. Take away memories and leave no scars.

Respect the animals. Learn from them. Appreciate with reverence the special places in which they dwell, their niches in a broader world and their individual meaning to you, the hunter.

And finally, respect yourself and your body. Care for it and it will take care of you, carrying you through spruce stands and cattail marshes and away from stressful situations. The healthy hunter emits an inner strength and confidence that cannot be bought nor given as a gift.

That's what this book is all about. It is about a process, a way of life, a way to extend your season throughout the years. And so as you think of autumn, "that aerobic time of year," inspire a little deeper and accelerate your heart rate a few beats. For the soul of autumn is October, a month with a pump up personality all its own. This book is an October kind of book. Smile a lot and sweat a bit.

Jeffry A. Metheny

Jeffry A. Metheny

Contents
The Meat of the Matter

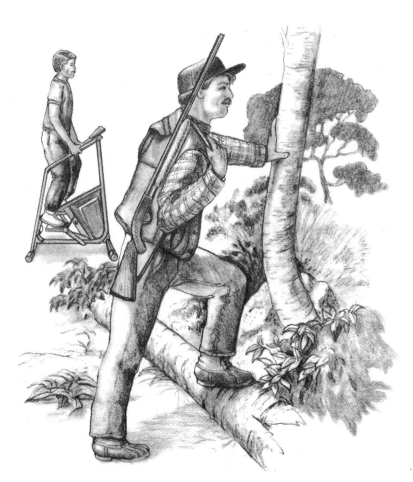

Chapter 1

The Hunter — The Athlete

When Frank Forester, Ernest Thompson Seaton and other literary godfather, American sportsmen first penned their sporting journals in the late 19th century, never could they have imagined the evolution of sports to the present day. To them, a sporting event was a day outdoors with a friend, be he human or

1

canine, enjoying all that nature had to offer. I seriously doubt that even in their most forethoughtful moments could they have imagined the World Series, domed football stadiums, or Olympic competition, let alone haggling over multi-million dollar contracts. How times have changed!

Heroes then were men who could scramble fast behind a pair of Gordon setters, shoot the lights out of a November sky, and spin adventure tales that held the local gentry spellbound. But sometime after the turn of century heroes changed. Then came the Ty Cobbs, Jack Dempseys and later Jesse Owens as ultimate sports role models. Attitudes were altered as well. These new men of sports grew in glamor and notoriety, no longer considering themselves sportsmen, but rather the elite upper crust known as athletes. The athlete viewed himself as a gifted individual blessed with natural ability and the determination to develop a highly specific skill in physical competition.

The age of the athlete was upon America and everyone wanted to partake of the dream. Like dandelions in April, athletic teams sprung up across the country. Men wore athletic supporters to feel more in step. Others developed nasty little fungus infections between their toes and swore that athletes alone were so priviledged to suffer this itching dermatitis. Times and attitudes continue to vascilate and grow, for now we are set on stamping out the athlete's foot fungus and not only do they wear them but now we actually refer to athletes as jocks.

And what has become of the sportsmen? What about the sportswomen and all of us who still enjoy the out-of-doors? We too, have grown and evolved, not as teams but as a large fraternity; not with glamor and glory but with an inner sense of appreciation and adventure. For some mysterious and unknown reason we still strongly feel the restless urgency of nature calling, especially when days grow short and mornings arise crisp and clear. We need our sport just as a tennis player needs a clay court, a golfer the long, green fairway, or a shortstop a well groomed infield. We need it for the thrill and excitement, the sense of accomplishment, and the serenity of quality time well spent.

The infamous and incorrigible market hunter is gone forever, however there still remain a significant number of professional guides and wildlife photographers that earn healthy incomes from stalking America's wildlife. To them, hunting remains a lifestyle that supports their families not just their fantasies and they must keep abreast of changes that might increase their proficiency.

Certain aspects of hunting have experienced healthy growth, particularly technological advances in equipment and clothing. We no longer need Long-Tom shotguns to deliver a black powder charge after a hurtling bird at 40 yards and compound bows have eliminated the serious drag and hold needed to launch an arrow with adequate force. Likewise, most of us no longer don heavy canvas oilskins in the drizzling dawn but now slip into well insulated Gortex parkas.

If attitude were a '55 Chevy however, hunters still often ride in the backseat of the sports world. Few consider themselves athletes or hunting a sports event. However if one analyzes the physical and mental components, requirements, and preparations, we see that hunting has many similarities to other recreational and even competitive athletics. No one can simply walk into their local sporting goods store, buy a shotgun, and wander off "hunting" anymore than one could purchase a set of golf clubs and consider himself a 4 handicap golfer, without ever having set a ball on a tee.

No matter whether you enjoy the sweat and hard work of a hunt, or merely a walk in the woods in search of game, hunting is a skill sport that requires background knowledge and physical effort. I remember well the late days of October scouring the New Hampshire hillside acres of aspen gold in search of woodcock with a professional mentor fifty years my senior. He was truly one of the old masters of orthopedics and he hit the brush behind his English setter with the same degree of vigor and proper purpose. Always dressed formally in his white broadcloth shirt with button down collars, tie and Filson vest, he would race toward his pointing Lady, screaming to get my attention. It was always "Dr. Metheny, Dr. Metheny, Point" in proper formality.

One dreary day after an amazing escapade of timberdoodle shooting during a sudden snow storm, he thoroughly surprised and confused me relating his admiration and amazement at how I carried myself in the woods. To me it was nothing more than careful cruising over fallen logs, around blackberry brambles and through white dogwood thickets; something I had grown up doing. But to a man who spent his first forty years in the city of Boston, it hadn't come that easily. He told me of moving to the White Mountains at age forty in search of a more durable and satisfying lifestyle, of becoming hypnotized and endeared to the migrating timberdoodle and most interestingly, how he had to learn to "walk in the woods". Something that I had taken for granted from my childhood excursions, he suffered through with twisted ankles, bruised shins, split lips and ears, not to mention the host of muscle strains and aching joints. And that was only part of the fun of learning to hunt doodles.

He also had to acquire knowledge of his game by reading books and magazines and experiencing the hunt with others who had been there before. That much came easily as an educational effort in studying the game, its habitat, and habits. The more difficult skills required included: reading cover, traversing unruly terrain, the flush, the swing, and the shot. After thirty autumns of chasing woodcock, he still found himself at times preoccupied with just how to circle a white pine or approach a vine covered understudy of an old apple tree while maintaining intense focus on the possible presence of a twittering woodcock or two. It is impossible to shoot well when you're preoccupied with keeping your feet on the ground.

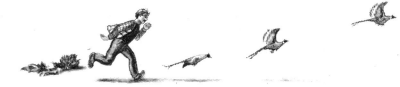

His experiences aroused my awareness that it took a special aptitude to be a successful hunter. Shooting ability is merely a small but important aspect of this aptitude. It can be improved by practicing on the trap or archery range during the off-season, as we all know. Between seasons most of us forget all about the physical aspects involved in hunting. If we could monitor your heart rate no doubt we'd discover the physical demands are usually excessive, as known by all who have tried to chase a running ringneck. To meet these demands, some degree of physical fitness and stamina are required and it is this major concept that most hunters have either forgotten or neglected to address.

Physical fitness awareness has flourished for the past decade or two. Numbers, though they may be surprising, speak truths. Each year, 50 million hunters take to the fields and forest across America in pursuit of their favorite game. By sheer number alone, hunting ranks high alongside swimming and walking as the most popular forms of physical exercise practiced in the United States.

When someone asks "Why do you exercise"?, the answers are many: "I exercise for competition, my mind, my health, or my heart". It could easily be said as well, "I exercise to hunt". Visualizing myself as an athlete and coupling this with my love for hunting, the "run to hunt" concept is an easy one to identify and grasp.

Physical fitness plays a major role in any sport for three basic reasons; performance, greater enjoyment of the event, and to lessen the risk of injury during the efforts of the event. For the athletic hunter performance is always important. When William Harndon Foster first developed skeet shooting, it was presumed to be the ideal practice to improve performance in grouse hunting. It helps no doubt, but how many times have you strolled leisurely down ten feet of concrete sidewalk, mounted your gun, yelled "Pull", shot and retrieved a downed partridge? You can see that skeet shooting provides only one aspect of practice necessary to be successful in the hill and dale tangles of grouse hunts.

Hunters are more like our Olympic biathletes, who cross country ski at top speed, stop suddenly, control their muscles and breathing to accurately shoot five targets before skiing off to repeat the task once again. Think then of a pheasant hunter in hot pursuit of his springer through chest high tule reeds, staying close to the action until finally the nervous bird erupts, and you see the similarity. Depending on the situation and conditions, some degree of physical fitness is important, so that our bodies move rapidly and respond physically and so we don't find ourselves trembling and out of breath, a limp scarecrow, when game finally presents itself. With respect to skeet shooting and simulating grouse hunting, not so, unless we are doing 30 yard dashes between shots. It is this combination of physical and shooting skills that makes the successful hunter.

Performance and goals are viewed differently by all and hunting companions are best chosen by matching these elements. We all know of a fitness fanatic who lifts weights every day and lives by his digital marathoner watch, pacing his feet while printing his pulse. For this occasional, obsessive hunter, a goal may be to cover ten miles before noon and if he gets a shot, well and good, but most of us don't enjoy racing through the woods and are not concerned what our split times are traversing a given terrain. By the same token and at the other extreme, hunting with the individual who can consistently break 24 out of 25 clay pigeons, but with similar consistency is out of breath and needs a break after a vigorous half mile walk, can be even more frustrating. My ideal companion will be an enthusiastic, average shot that can stay after game all day rather than the target splitters who constantly need to regather and recoup.

Hunting, more than any other sport, abides by the adage, "It's not winning or losing but how you play the game". Hunting is not measured merely by performance nor success by obtaining your limit. The enjoyment felt from a day afield, away from concrete, cars, and the mundane routines is heightened by physical fitness. The sky, royal blue; air, crisp and chilled; the mosiac of autumn colors and the leathery smell of aspen and oak are appreciated fully without concern of running out of gas halfway up a hill or the anxiety of how long you can hold your bow at full draw.

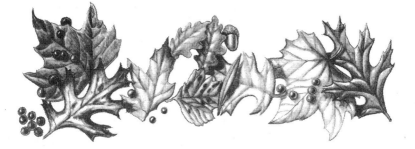

When you have prepared yourself for the season, you approach it with confidence and security and now are more able to focus on reading cover, relating to the nuances of your new Brittany, and being attentive to your reaction time when game is sighted.

Knowing that your body can meet the physical demands alleviates anxiety and preoccupations about keeping up, whether your heart will stop, or how terrible you will feel in the morning. Preparing your body for the upcoming season as other athletes do, improves not only performance but also the perception of the hunt.

Each of us has experienced at least one year when time was short and September simply snuck up on us. Remembering with boyhood hindsight, a time when we could walk all day, lugging grandpa's ten pound Remington and not miss a beat, we spring out of our all too sedentary existance and hit the hills with vigor. That day usually is one to remember and makes for one long and frustrating season, not to speak of bone weary Mondays and minor aches and pains that continually remind you that you are either growing older, out of shape, or more likely both. The final aspect that the athlete-hunter concept addresses is one of injury prevention and treatment. Nothing frustrates and angers a hunter more than spending hours planning, saving money for the hunt of the season, or perhaps even the hunt of a lifetime, only to pull a calf muscle or develop knee tendinitis the first day out and have the entire trip ruined.

The specialty of sportsmedicine recognizes that athletes are different and therefore require a different philosophy and treatment format. Athletes have a sense of urgency with a very short time frame. Their physical requirements as well as the injuries they suffer form patterns that are specifically dependent on the sport that they engage. In most sports, patterns have been researched extensively and sportsmedicine literature is replete with magazine articles and even entire books directed toward recreational and competitive athletes participating in conventional sports, but for the hunter very few guidelines are available. There is no question that hunters suffer similar patterns of injuries, many of which overlap into other sports and some are specific to hunting alone. Identifying these injuries, the persons at risk and by addressing them with preventive and rehabilitative concepts, hunting season no longer has to be approached feeling "no pain, no gain".

Overuse injuries are common and quickly and easily forgotten if our daily routine involves limited physical activity but they also dessimate an entire hunt where one needs daily strength and endurance over miles of rugged walking. Strains and sprains of the muscles, bones, and joints can be prevented, or at least lessened, by a preseason fitness program. Research evidence has proven that a well conditioned musculoskeletal system reacts more rapidly, is less prone to injury, and is more resilient to repetitive stresses resulting in less exercise induced soreness. Well conditioned bones and joints are also less likely to sprain ligaments when rapidly torqued or suffer stress fractures which are micro failures of the bone due to repeated overuse.

The need for physical conditioning can be best appreciated by individuals who have suffered through previous injuries and those who have acquired arthritis. These people are acutely aware of their need for exercise conditioning to prevent further damage and wear on their already abnormal joints. The ideal goal of sportsmedicine is to prevent injuries rather than to fix the ones that have already occurred.

Softball players, runners, golfers, and hunters, we are all athletes of a type. It is only our sport that differs. The concept of the athlete-hunter focuses us on conditioning and preparation so that we can improve our performance, prevent, or at least limit, our physical injuries, and most important, enjoy our hunting season maximally.

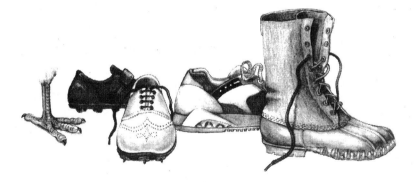

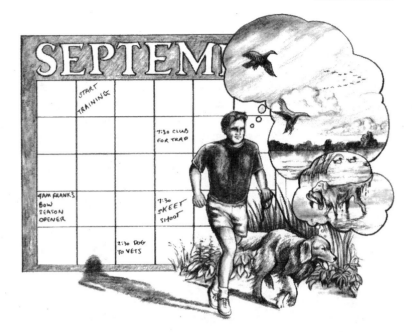

Chapter 2

Preseason Conditioning
September's Song of Effort

E very major and most minor sports today require some type of
preseason preparation. Baseball has its spring training and
football its summer camps. The goal of this preparation is not only
to select members of the team and practice to improve performance
but also to make a final push to prepare the body for its upcoming
use and abuse during the rapidly approaching season. The moans
and groans that echo through these training camps speak loudly of
bodies out of shape, and of bodies being pushed beyond normal
physical effort, but in time the straining and aching subside as
these bodies adapt to their new demands.

After all is said, conditioning is adaptation and therein lies one
flexible beauty of the human body. Given a physical task, and

repeating it until the task has been completed with satisfaction, the various body systems (particularly the cardiovascular and musculo-skeletal) grow accustomed to what is being asked of them. Gradually the task becomes less of an effort, less of a strain, more fluid and coordinated and usually more enjoyable. That's not to say that everyone can win one Tour de France or play nose tackle for the Chicago Bears, but we all can be better than we are. It takes time, preparation and a healthy dose of perspiration. For the pro or the athletic hunter, preseason conditioning is a key concept to enhance enjoyment, performance, and lessen the risk of injury.

When should training begin? In times past an X on the calendar marked the opening of the season and if time allowed the weekend before, the dog was loaded into the back of the stationwagon and driven to local park or sportsmen's club to limber up and work out some kinks that might have developed over the past nine months of infrequent exercise. After an hour or so of strolling, the dog and master pile back into the stationwagon, out of breath, and still fostering a few glaring misconceptions. First and foremost is that this bit of preseason exercise was for the dog alone and it was he that needed to toughen his paws, suck a little wind and drop a few pounds. The other misconstrued thought was that an hour, a day, or even a week can shake out the physical wrinkles that have formed over months of inactivity. One goal of this book is to try to dispel old myths, to change habits and to interject new ideas that benefit hunters not just from October to December but all year. The hope is a lifestyle change for the love of hunting and the desire to continue the sport for many future seasons. This means the calendar is open and conditioning ongoing. Ideally then, preseason should really be offseason, a year-round program with increased intensity in the later summer as the season draws nigh.

Sports research has shown that for the average 25 to 45 year old male it takes four to six weeks of structured conditioning to get one's body into shape. For the older individual or those who are planning very physically taxing trips, the training period will obviously be longer.

Before embarking on a vigorous exercise program, the first step for those over forty years of age is a visit to your family physician for an "annual" physical examination, perhaps your first "annual" exam in 15 years. The doctor will recognize those individuals who are at high risk for heart attacks. For high risk persons this examination should include a stress electrocardiogram. This type of EKG is a monitored recording of your heart, before, during and after a bout of serious exercise, running on a treadmill or riding an exercise bike. It provides the physician with information about how your heart responds and performs when subjected to physical stress. It is a much more accurate method to see just how your heart will act when you are excitedly racing after a downed pheasant in thick cover or hauling your whitetail buck up a steep, half-mile logging road.

People considered high risk are those who have a family history or personal history of heart attacks in the past, those who have had recent chest pain, smokers, or people with high blood pressure, and finally those who live sedentary lifestyles. Anything sound familiar? It is also a wise precaution to have your blood cholesterol measured for an abnormally high cholesterol (above 250 total count) can be a silent but dangerous risk indicator. Explain to your physician what your goals are; he will be better able to evaluate your general medical condition and specifically the status of your heart. Nothing, and I mean nothing, will ruin a hunt let alone end your life like a heart attack.

To simplify a conditioning program one should think of three basic areas to exercise; cardiovascular, musculoskeletal and activity specific training. Each of these areas must be addressed so the entire body gradually adapts to the physical stress and demands of the sport.

Cardiovascular conditioning refers to exercise specifically directed at the heart. The heart, being the most vital muscle of the body, works together with the lungs to provide oxygen-rich blood to all body parts. Just like every muscle in the body, the heart will adapt to a gradual, progressive exercise program to increase its endurance and response to increased demands.

The concept of aerobic exercise became popular in the 1970's when medical studies demonstrated the beneficial effects of aerobically conditioning all muscles, specifically the heart and also the relationship of this exercise form to preventing coronary artery disease. Aerobic conditioning does not refer only to a roomful of bouncing women wearing tights, exercising to the beat of a popular dance tune, but in its scientifically broad sense refers to a prolonged, low intensity exercise, using the larger muscles of the trunk, the arms and legs. Further the term aerobic relates to the heavy breathing and oxygen intake while performing certain exercise and even more specifically to a very particular enzyme pathway in all muscles that is turned on when the muscle functions continuously for at least twenty minutes. Therefore to reach an aerobic level, the exercise must involve large muscles and be performed continuously for that length of time. Thus, it is not as simple as flushing the pipes, but when the heart muscle is stressed aerobically, its function improves on a cellular and biochemical level as well.

For your heart to obtain aerobic benefit its rate must be increased to a point where it is pumping at 60% to 80% of its maximum capacity. This maximum capacity as measured in beats per minute varies with age and can be quickly calculated by taking 220 and subtracting your age. For example a forty year old male's maximum heart rate is 180. To achieve an aerobic level of activity to benefit his heart he must exercise to reach a pulse rate of 108 to 144 beats per minute. Pulse can be monitored during exercise at the carotid artery along the side of the neck, or at the radial artery on the thumb side of the wrist. Further cardiovascular studies have shown that to maximize the benefit to the heart and help prevent heart attack, aerobic activity must be done at least three times a week.

As a brief summary, cardiovascular conditioning requires physical exercise to obtain a heart rate of 60% to 80% of maximum. The physical effort is continued for at least 20 minutes and must be repeated at least three times a week. Common aerobic activities include jogging or rapid walking, swimming, bicycling, cross country skiing, and rowing. For the beginner the aerobic exercise should be started at five to ten minute intervals and increased approximately five minutes per week. An aggressive hunter will want to increase his endurance and stamina by exercising for an hour or more. It has also been shown that continuing aerobic exercise beyond a 30 minute time interval greatly increases the mobilization and utilization of the body's fat stores in providing energy. Therefore if weight loss is a preseason goal as well, aerobic type activities for 30 to 60 minutes will greatly enhance weight reduction.

For those with prior injuries or arthritis, the majority of your aerobic training can be done with as little impact loading and stress on the joints as possible. Low impact aerobic activities such as biking, swimming, cross country ski machines, and steppers are becoming more popular.

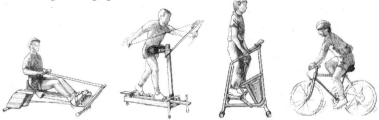

Musculoskeletal conditioning is an area with which most of us are quite familiar and centers around muscle flexibility or stretching and resistance exercise or weight lifting. The key concept to grasp is that hunting, like most forms of athletic and recreational endeavors does not require a great deal of strength but does involve many repetitions with submaximal effort, better known as endurance. We don't sprint after a deer nor do we wrestle with a bear. We do walk briskly for many miles, often carrying an eight pound rifle in our arms, two to three pounds of boots on our feet and five to fifteen pounds wrapped snugly around our trunk in our vest. Thus, when we discuss weight lifting it will be weight training with multiple repetitions at lower weights rather than power lifting for ultimate strength.

Another important physiological point is that warmed-up muscles are more flexible, resilient, and responsive muscles. Joints and muscles that are stressed excessively while cold will more likely be stiff and sore and prone to strains throughout the day. Body temperature is maintained close to 98.6 degrees Fahrenheit but the joint and muscle temperature can be raised a degree or so by repeated gentle contractions or by stretching. Stretching, or flexibility, is a concern not only in preseason conditioning but throughout the season and of particular importance the morning before a hunt. When was the last time you visited a deer camp when everybody bailed out of bed five minutes early to stretch out and warm up? Did you ever hear the camp cook counting off jumping jacks as his bacon sizzled? But then again, when was the time you last visited a deer camp that was without its share of aches, pains, and moans and groans? Hunters bounce out of bed the first morning, then crawl out thereafter. It doesn't have to be like that.

Flexibility training, stretching, doesn't take long. Each group of muscles should be isolated and held in a stretched manner for thirty seconds for maximum benefit, not in the bouncing or jarring fashion that many of us learned in our high school physical education classes. Slow and steady gets you ready!

Develop a routine starting with the head and progress toward the toes. The neck should be bent forward and held for 30 seconds, backwards and held, (Figure 2-1A) and subsequently to each side, (Figure 2-1B) and rotating or looking over each shoulder. Neck circles involve complex movement, don't sustain adequate stretch, often aggravate neck pain and therefore should be avoided.

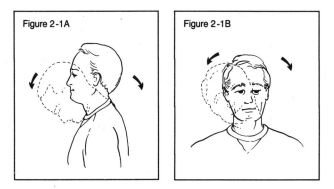

Figure 2-1A   Figure 2-1B

Stretching the back can be done by toe touches, both together or alternating sides, thus rotating the back while bending forward (Figure 2-2). Back extensions involve arching the low back to a comfortable position and holding for 30 seconds (Figure 2-3) and are excellent for those prone to disk problems.

Muscles in the legs are the ones most often affected by overuse injuries such as strains and tendinitis, so a few extra minutes here are warranted. The quadriceps (front thigh muscle group) are stretched by standing, facing or even holding onto a wall or chair for balance, reaching behind your body, grasping your foot and then gently pulling your foot towards your bottom and drawing the

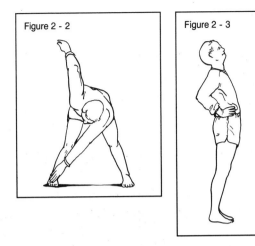

Figure 2 - 2

Figure 2 - 3

knee backwards away from the wall (Figure 2-4). The hamstrings, (back thigh muscles) are stretched by doing toe touches, remembering not to "bounce" or by modified hurdler's stretches, putting one foot on a chair, counter or low stool, keeping the knee straight and then leaning downward toward your leg (Figure 2-5).

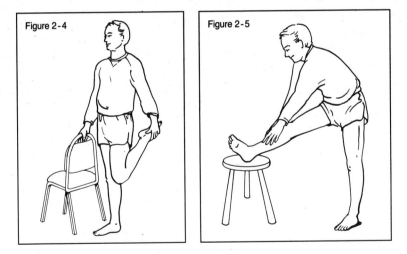

Figure 2-4

Figure 2-5

Calf muscle stretches are performed facing a wall, an arm's length away with feet spread slightly apart. Both hands should be placed on the wall, both heels on the ground and the knees should be kept straight initially while you lean toward the wall and hold for a 30 second count (Figure 2-6A). This should then be repeated with both knees bent 20 to 30 degrees (Figure 2-6B) to stretch lower calf and foot muscles. This stretch may also be done alternating one straight and one bent knee.

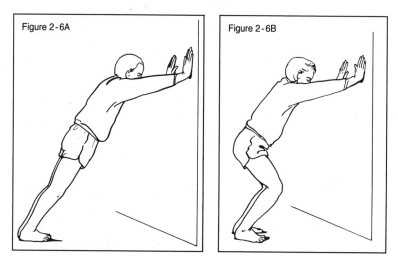

Figure 2-6A

Figure 2-6B

Elbows and shoulders are very mobile joints, inherently flexible, rarely requiring stretching exercises unless they have been injured.

This entire flexibility routine of slow, sustained stretching of each major muscle group for at least 30 seconds takes about 5-10 minutes. If you have ever wondered why all the warm-ups before major athletic events, it is to prepare the muscles and joints for rapid response during the game and also to prevent injuries.

Resistance exercises or weight training may be less important than flexibiity to those afield, unless you anticipate a long drag of your 200 pound 10 point buck or lengthy hike back up a draw lugging a 25 pound tom turkey. Weight training can be looked at as adjunctive exercise to improve reaction time and speed of response. Perhaps more importantly it also improves the muscles shock absorption capability so that the many hard miles of walking and climbing do not strain muscles or damage joints. Strong resilient muscles act much like the springs and shocks of an automobile, thereby preventing undue wear on the wheels. Toning muscles also improves response time. For example; how fast, how often and how smoothly you swing your 12 gauge on flocks of ducks throughout an entire day depends on the durability of repeated muscle contraction. Obviously both strength and endurance are necessary in certain types of hunting, such as the bow hunter repeatedly shooting an 80 pound compound.

Whereas upper extremity weight lifting may be optional, leg strengthening is mandatory to improve your ability to walk all day, climb up and down hills and of course protect your ligaments and joints from injuries such as sprained knees or ankles.

The quadriceps is the key muscle in the leg and so goes the quad, so goes the hunt. Strengthening it is done by sitting on a chair or a counter top with weights inserted into a knapsack or purse dangling over the ankle. One may also purchase commercially made ankle weights with velcro fasteners that can be wrapped comfortably about the ankle. Starting from a flexed position the knee is gradually extended until straight and held for five seconds (Figure 2-7). Maximum strength benefits require a five second hold on each lift and 10 consecutive lifts or repetitions. Ideally you would lift three to four sets of 10 repetitions, one leg at a time. Starting light with five pounds one can progress weekly by 5 to 10 pounds up to 30 pounds with one leg—higher weights may actually put too much force on the kneecap and cause pain. So if you feel a need for further exertion, increase the number of repetitions rather than the weight itself. The use of Universal Gym, Nautilus or other exercise equipment is optional. Jogging and

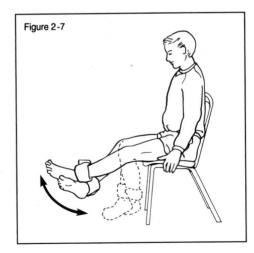

Figure 2-7

bicycling build quad strength too. Proper strengthening of the quadriceps is the most effective way to prevent tendinitis of the knee and pain about the kneecap so commonly seen after hill climbing.

Toe raises, with or without weights, strengthen the calf and foot muscles, add bounce to the step, and help prevent Achille's tendinitis and calf cramps. Use a five second hold at the top of your raise and do three to four sets of 10 repetitions. To maximize strengthening, increase the number of repetitions, wear a weighted vest or simply do single legged toe raises (Figure 2-8). Rope jumping is an excellent activity—not only to strengthen the calf muscles but also improve agility and balance, important properties when cruising the woods on a slick morning.

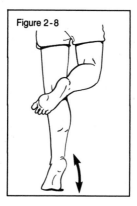

Figure 2-8

The last area to be covered by a preseason conditioning program is directed by the demands of a specific activity, simply what kind of hunting you will be doing. Activity specific exercise takes some thought and analysis of the type of hunting, gear, terrain, duration of the hunt and desired pace. Consider the duration, the intensity, and terrain of the hunt, such as an all-out, no holds-barred, five day hunt for British Columbia Dall sheep. Training requirements dictate high intensity work-outs in high altitude mountains with packing gear and many weeks of advance preparation. These Dall sheep hunters' requirements differ entirely from the Klamath River chukar shooter in hot dry weather chasing after his normally obedient German Shorthair. Each hunter must analyze the demands of the upcoming hunt and direct your preparation specifically for it, being as innovative as possible.

In doing so, you don't dispense with nor forget your general cardiovascular and musculoskeletal system training but rather use your general conditioning to help achieve a certain goal. This is the concept of cross-training. It is only by your extra work on flexibility and strengthening that you can concentrate on more precise exercise objectives.

Exercise is quite specific in the results it produces. You become a good hockey player by playing hockey. The stretching and weight lifting will help but not like actually playing the game or participating in exercise that closely simulates the sport. Not to understate the obvious, you cannot climb off an exercise bicycle even if you have been riding for an hour a clip and expect to scale rocky peaks with a 20 pound pack. After your hunt analysis, try to locate similar terrain in your locale, don your gear or an equivalent thereof, "loading a knapsack or vest with weights, carrying hand weights, etc", climb up and down or slog the marsh. Only then will you know specificity. Only then will you really be truly conditioned and feel your body adapted for specific demands ahead. Incorporating the information in this and other chapters a weekly program can be designed to prepare you for opening day. A three day cycle appeals to most.

Day #1	Flexibility training	10 minutes
	Low impact aerobics	30-60 minutes
Day #2	Flexibility training	10 minutes
	Weight training	60 minutes
Day #3	Rest	

As the season approaches substitute one day of weight lifting per week with a day of sport specific training.

Everyone is aware of the need to practice and that practice brings skill improvement. Simply visiting the trap range for a few nights the week before the season starts is grossly underestimating need and forgetful of what the majority of hunting is all about. Much more time is spent on physical effort than aiming a gun. Hours of precious, patient perspiration are spent on each 5 second shot. Preseason conditioning demands discipline and hard work and certainly more than running a few rounds through the chamber. The athlete hunter must be both gradual with his progression and consistent in his exercise program but ultimately it will improve his performance, heighten his enjoyment, and prevent injuries.

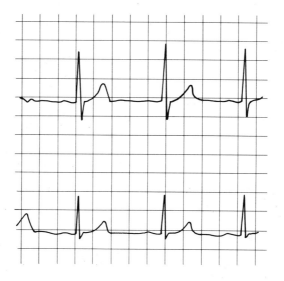

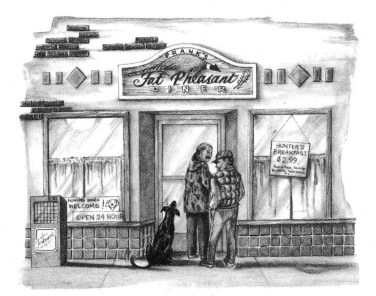

Chapter 3

The Institution of Breakfast
The Ham and Eggs of Hunting

Hunting is a sport of rituals; from checklist preparation and selection of gear, placing decoys out in one particular set, to following the same trail to your deer stand at precisely the same time as you have each year since you bagged "Old Stealthy". Very few traditions however become so ingrained as the prehunt breakfast. For some unknown reason, most spouses don't share the same degree of enthusiasm that hunters do in regard to food preparation at 4 AM. Therefore we have come to rely on the infamous "camp cook" or local eateries that cater to our early morning appetite.

As he has for many years, the designated camp cook arises in the predawn. He is a veteran of many seasons and now has accepted the charge of filling up his sleeping, soon to arise companions with lots of stick to the rib vittles and gallons of coffee to wash away the early morning cobwebs and crank over the old engine. The bacon slab is soon spitting, toast heavily buttered and as the yawns of his companions fill the cabin like those of a family of grizzlies sharing one hibernation cave, dozens of eggs drop onto the griddle and lay there sputtering. Nothing like it! How many eggs, 3-4? Sure! Add more bacon and toast. It is cold out there and you need to feed your boilers. Wiping our mouths, we push away from the table, stuffed, complacent and ready to sack out for a few more hours. Camp cooks are rare legacies.

Many of us are not so fortunate to have been associated with such a colorful charactor, he either having passed on, or simply quit such a thankless chore. There still however remains the local diner, the one that either stays open all night or opens its doors at ungodly morning hours to corner the market on sleepy hunters. The decor may run from Early American railroad car, or primitive pioneer log lodge to original fifties funk, but some items remain consistent. They each will have a jukebox full of old Elvis and recent Willie Nelson, the faint aroma of Camel cigarettes and smoked ham, coffee served in thick ceramic mugs so hot your lips singe and a no-nonsense waitress that knows how to get the job done. The menu likewise remains relatively constant, as sausages and omelettes are shoveled rapidly into gaping mouths and then in a flash it's off to the nearby marsh for early morning exercise and excitement chasing ringnecks through the cattails. Stepping out of the truck your legs feel leadened, your body moves slowly and the heaviness in your stomach is obvious. You'd rather be facing your bunk or sleeping bag than the mudsucking march that lies ahead.

Far be it from me to even consider such a sacrilegious act as denouncing something as American as ham and eggs, but the old idea of sticking the ribs full of heavy, fatty foods simply doesn't hold water. Such breakfasts smell devine, taste fantastic, but this type of eating does create some basic problems for the hunter. We all know that high fat and high cholesterol diets have long term implications in the narrowing of coronary arteries, thus increasing the risk of heart attacks, but we are not talking or even thinking long term now. We are concerned with the immediate and subsequent effects of how your body responds to this intake throughout the day.

It is true that gram for gram fats contain much higher energy (calories—9:1) than either proteins or carbohydrates. So in a starvation situation fats are highly desireable but rarely does anyone find themselves concerned with survival nor that far from food. Usually the problem is quite the opposite. It is also true that fats are much more difficult to digest and large loads tend to make the body sluggish, even hours after eating. Fats will also remain in the stomach longer and may cause abdominal discomfort, bloating and cramping with exercise. Thus, eating a meal high in fat content just prior to physical activity is setting one's body up for unnecessary and uncomfortable feelings.

The best alternative energy source prior to physical exertion is carbohydrates in the form of cereals, pastas, breads, and rice. Carbohydrates digest easily and are absorbed into the blood as readily useable energy sources in less than half the time of fat. In keeping with the athlete-hunter theme, dinner the night before the hunt should be high in carbohydrate much like marathon runners' carbohydrate loading meal to maximize the body's accessible energy stores. A dinner of spaghetti and bread provides this readily available energy more so than steak and baked potatoes smothered in butter and sour cream. Likewise, a breakfast of pancakes, waffles, muffins, cereal, and fruit could substitute nicely for foods high in fat. You will be able to peak and maintain a higher level of energy and endurance with this type of high carbohydrate breakfast. You also won't be troubled by after breakfast sluggishness so common after a fatty meal.

Throughout a strenuous day of hunting it is necessary to replenish energy stores with a light lunch or occasional snacks. I will never forget one well known outdoor writer a few years ago recommending his readers try his favorite high energy sandwich for lunch; bread filled with cream cheese, peanut butter, and six strips of bacon—be assured that eating a sandwich like that would cement one to the spot and require an after dinner nap for an hour or so. Definitely loads of calories and most of them fat and cholesterol. Again, it is best to avoid foods with heavy fatty (triglyceride and cholesterol) content and make your sandwiches of light cheese, chicken or turkey. Snacks of crackers, cookies and fruit will also provide and sustain your energy throughout the day without you experiencing a bogged down period.

Some individuals are prone to episodic hypoglycemia or low blood sugar. This phenomenon occurs in people with insulin imbalance (opposite of diabetes), or even in normal individuals after heavy physical activity and usually comes on in mid afternoon if you haven't eaten anything for hours. The depletion of the body's energy stores without replenishment presents signs of hypoglycemia. The hunter may feel dizziness, shaking, weakness, experience poor coordination and at times, when severe, even sweating and confusion. Any of these symptoms warrant a quick sugar load such as candy, gum, or cookies, and realization that the day is late and you should think about returning home for further nutritional intake.

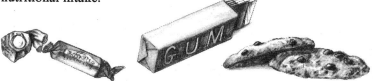

Dehydration or fluid depletion, can also create similar feelings of dizziness and shaking but you will feel very thirsty. Your body will tell you it is dry and crave fluids, but often there is a time lag between actual depletion and symptoms. When hunting, frequent stops for rehydration are mandatory and on a given day a hunter will require between two to four gallons of water, depending on the day's temperature and humidity as well as the intensity of the exercise.

Don't equate sweat with the need to drink. In dry, windy climates, perspiration may not be apparent when in reality body water losses through sweat evaporation is usually tremendous. Even in cold weather body water loss can be quite high for much body water is lost during heavy respiration when exercising. It is a wise and comfortable hunter that carries a canteen or water bottle in his vest if drinking water from springs or streams is not otherwise readily accessible. Newly marketed fanny packs or velcro belt and water bottle systems that carry water for ultra-marathoners and triathletes offer an ideal way to transport fluids without realizing added weight. They ride close to your body and don't impede mounting your gun.

What you carry in your thermos or drinking container is also important. Drinks that are heavily sweetened can actually increase your thirst. Plain water is still the best replacement fluid and best satisfies the sensation of thirst. Electrolyte solutions so common at sporting events are unnecessary as the body's ability to autoregulate and maintain electrolyte balance in the blood is remarkable. The small amount of simple sugars they contain can however give you a quick boost later in the day.

Caffeine drinks such as tea, coffee, cola, as well as alcohol are diuretics and theoretically stimulate the kidneys to excrete more water with an overall effect of further dehydration, so don't assume that you can adequately rehydrate yourself with coffee or beer. (Reason number 327 why alcohol and hunting don't mix.)

Remember to drink before you are thirsty, for once the body senses thirst, the body is dehydrated approximately two to three percent of your total body weight and it takes quite some time to replace and recover. The best tactic is to drink small amounts every 30 to 60 minutes throughout the day rather than one to two quarts at one sitting. Again, sip and sip frequently. One other way that explorers and mountaineers have monitored their state of hydration is by noting the color of their urine. Normal urine should be very lightly tinged with yellow. Very simply, the lighter and clearer the urine the better the hydration and conversely the darker yellow urine means the kidneys are retaining as much water as possible, allowing the darker waste products to be excreted. Dark urine means you need some fluid.

We have been told for ages that we are what we eat and to a degree there is a certain amount of truth in that statement. There is no doubt that an exercising athlete's day is best started with a filling, high carbohydrate and relatively low fat breakfast, followed by similar light lunch and snacks throughout the day. Keep the mid-afternoon blahs so commonly caused by hypoglycemia or dehydration away by frequent and intermittently snacking and drinking water. If you must retain tradition and gorge yourself, do it at the evening meal, hopefully partaken at least two hours before bedtime so your digestive tract doesn't remind you all night about each and every bite you had for dinner — If you don't believe you are what you eat, at least believe you dream what you eat.

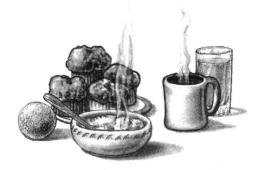

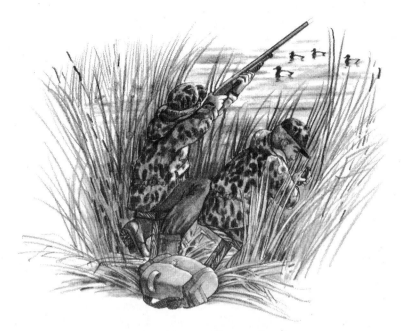

Chapter 4

Back to the Blind

He pressed the accelerator a little closer to the floor just as the stoplight turned yellow. He is late. Although only 10 or 15 minutes behind schedule, he feels the pressure and knows his brother will be pacing the front porch in his waders anxiously sipping a cup of steaming coffee. He will be surrounded by duffle bags and decoys and wondering if his ride might just make it sometime before daybreak. This annual migration to the north shores of Lake Michigan in search of big breasted mallards, and if luck would have it, a few snows and Canadas, always creates some degree of urgent anxiety even if there is unlimited time for preparation. As usual, most of the effort for this trip came last night when clothes, calls, and all were slam-dunked into duffle bags, guns oiled and cased, waders checked for holes, camouflage netting folded, thermoses filled and decoys inspected and finally stowed in their net backpacks.

On the porch by the darkness of a new moon, the awaiting sibling reviews his mental checklist again for the 32nd time in 48 hours. Shells! How many boxes for this five day hunt, 5, 6? No, better take seven, in case big brother is forgetful this year.

The truck headlights swing across the grey-green lumps lying sprawled out on the porch. He sees the 16 foot flat tied to the truck roof has a new coat of camouflage. The brothers quickly exchange greetings and as quietly as possible load the bags, the packs, and at least another ton of necessary items into the back of an already crowded pick-up and steal away into the moonless night. It is 3 AM and a winding two hour drive will bring them to the lake shores and nearby flooded swamps and corn fields, that will hopefully be loaded with waterfowl.

As the driver crawls behind the steering wheel, he jerks and jitters trying to find a more comfortable sitting position. His back seems a bit stiff from all the packing last night and the black magic of loading two tons into a ¾ ton pickup. They stop at Frank's—Thanks For Stopping By, their favorite all night diner for a quick breakfast. Again, the stiffness grabs him when getting out of the truck but by the time they reach Frank's door he is able to straighten up and walk normally. Frank's—Thanks For Stopping By is an institution of incredible surprises, not so much the 1950 decor, nor the quality of food, but rather the quantity and amazing speed with which it magically appears in front of you. It disappears wth similar haste.

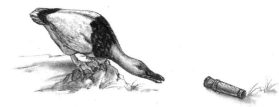

Back in the truck they drive the final hour, practicing mallard chuckles, widgeon squeaks, and woody whistles. Bumping slowly through water filled pot holes along the last two miles of gravel road they finally arrive at the DNR station, check in just in time to luckily draw a dynamite area for the morning's hunt. A brief drive down the old dike road to a deserted remnant of a parking lot and then the fun begins.

First the boat, a very substantial and stable old Herters' model is untied from the roof-top carrier and with a customary grunt and groan, lowered to the ground. Shotguns, shells, food and thermoses, raingear, camo netting, oars, life preservers, wooden stools and decoys "Ah, yes the decoys" are pulled out of the pickup bed and loaded into the flat.

"Where the Hell did all these decoys come from?"

"Well, I brought a dozen extra remembering those snow geese that flew by last year that we no doubt would have easily taken if we would have had a few white blocks out".

"Okay, I admit I brought a couple of dozen teal decoys for good luck."

The old warrior of a boat, only 16 feet long and three feet wide, was loaded to look more like an Erie canal barge. There was little room to ride so with waders and low water conditions they pushed and slid along the side of the DNR corn field out to their designated shooting area. Wade as rapidly as they might (aerobic sloshing), it still took 20 minutes to reach the spot for a makeshift blind. Even with both throwing decoys as quickly as a pair of excited Las Vegas dealers, daybreak had broken and the wings of mallard and teal already filled the skies. On a dead run, or should we say slosh, they pull the flat back into the corn rows, cover it with netting, grab guns, shells and stools and make their way to a clump of corn stalks fronting the decoys and with the wind at their backs. Plunging their marsh stools (basically a four foot length of 2 × 4's sharpened at one end, and with a 2″ × 8″ nailed to the other) solidly into the muck, they finally sit down tediously balanced on their unsteady seats, drenched with perspiration and panting for air. In time the dampness drys, the heavy breathing normalizes and now, the excitement of the wait.

For a bluebird morning, the ducks had moved well, answering to the call and they had picked up four drakes, two greenwings and a great Canada that just happened by and all this by 10 AM. Gradually the excitement of the wait evaporated simultaneously with the early sky's waterfowl. The intensity of the hunt is directly proportional to the number of ducks in the sky and as the excitement gradually disappears along with the morning flights, the mind turns to mundane things like a sandwich, a mug of coffee and Oh! there's that back pain again.

It seems whenever he sits or bends over too long, such as crouching motionless to prevent flaring oncoming flocks, the stiffness and aching occur. As the day progresses it becomes a little more uncomfortable slouching down to call and a bit slower and stiffer rising to shoot. By noon his back is telling him to get up and stretch, take a walk, and it's time to pick up and leave anyway. The boat is once again loaded, hauled back to the truck, unloaded and lifted atop. Who said duck hunting was easy, a leisurely stroll to a comfortable chair in some cozy blind? They arrive back at the DNR shed just in time for the afternoon drawing assignments and then begins the repetition of the morning's activities which seem more like work this time.

The evening star has risen high by the time they turn right into the Wild Goose Inn, a trusted local motel catering to duck hunters of all ages, at all times of the day. The moist evening air cooled considerably as they stiffly unpacked and carried their bag limits around back to a designated dressing area behind the motel. It consisted of a dim 60 watt light, a trash barrel, a faucet with four feet of hose and a 3 × 3 plywood slab on the ground. After an hour of bending and picking and bending and cleaning his back was really agonizing and some pain shot down the back of his left leg. Not a good way to start a five day waterfowl interlude.

Lumbago, the old nemesis called by many names including "My damn backache" has ruined many good times in the past and will continue to do so in the future.

This is a common saga of a man anxious to get away from his busy schedule, pressing himself into physical demands which his back simply isn't ready to tolerate. He has been so busy at work he has not had time to do his back exercises. Yet here he is loading and unloading tons of gear then adding insult to injury by subsequently sitting crouched and slumped in an unsupported seat all day, no doubt the worst of all worlds for his back. It is not at all difficult to predict the outcome.

Back pain is an enigma and no one has all the answers as to why it occurs or to whom. Low back aches can be due to: muscle strain or overuse of the low back muscles, arthritis or pinching of the small joints known as lumbar facets, or because of a disk slip or rupture.

A "slipped disk" usually presents itself in two different ways; one when there is an acute and complete herniation of the disk which pushes on a small nerve root, sending electric shocks down the leg, known as sciatica. More commonly however the disk will merely bulge back toward the nerve root and cause a nagging, toothache-like pain in the back and sometimes into the buttocks. This gradual process, known as degenerative disk disease is a function of aging and years of accumulative micro-trauma to the disks. Disks usually bulge or herniate at the fourth or fifth lumbar

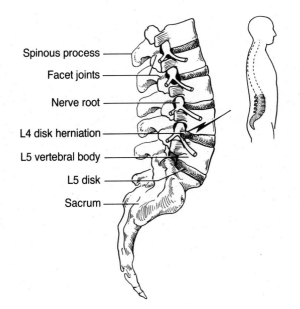

Spinous process
Facet joints
Nerve root
L4 disk herniation
L5 vertebral body
L5 disk
Sacrum

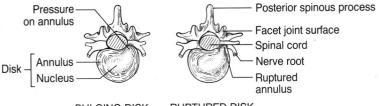

TOP VIEW OF LUMBAR VERTEBRAE

Pressure on annulus
Posterior spinous process
Facet joint surface
Spinal cord
Disk — Annulus
Nucleus
Nerve root
Ruptured annulus

BULGING DISK   RUPTURED DISK

vertebral level. Scientific studies have confirmed what many duck hunters have felt for ages, that activities placing increased pressure on the disk are bending over and lifting or sitting in a slouched position without a back support.

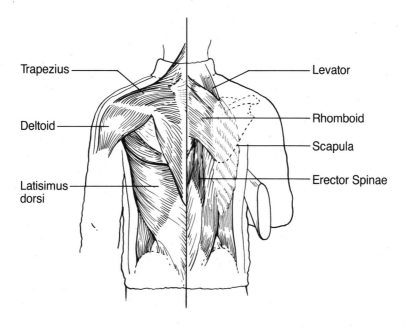

This scenario sounds familiar I'm sure, for more than 85% of Americans will see a doctor for back pain at some time in their life. People who have had this uncomfortable but common experience need to be on a preventive back care program which includes body weight control, knowledge of the biomechanics of lifting, ("how and how not to"), and special exercises to increase flexibility and balance out the back and abdominal muscles. This exercise program should include hamstring and back stretches, pelvic tilts, partial sit-ups, elbow props and press-ups.

Stretching is done lying on your back, bending your hip and holding one knee with your hands, bringing it up towards your chest (Figure 4-1). This knee to chest stretch should be done alternating the legs and finally bringing both legs up together simultaneously. Hamstring muscles in the back of the thigh are stretched either by a hurdler's maneuver or by lying flat on your back, keeping the knee straight and bringing the leg up towards your head (Figure 4-2). The exerciser may wrap his hands around behind his knee to keep the leg straight and to provide extra manual stretching.

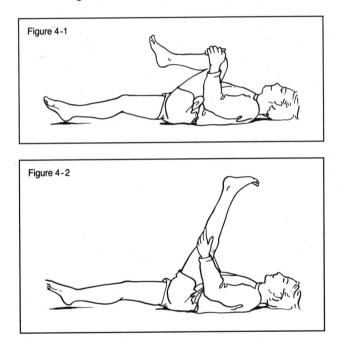

Figure 4-1

Figure 4-2

Pelvic tilts are performed, again lying on your back, with your knees bent and your feet on the floor. The upward arch of the low back is then consciously forced down toward the floor by tightening the abdominal muscles and rotating the pelvis forward, thereby creating a flat back (Figure 4-3). Partial sit-ups or crunches tone the abdominal muscles and are done, in a lying, bent-knee position, placing your hands behind your head or out to the side. A sit-up is initiated, merely clearing the shoulder blades from the floor and this is held for five seconds (Figure 4-4). Twenty-five to fifty partial sit-ups should be done daily. There is no need to sit completely upright into a full sit-up which actually creates increased pressure on the back and can aggravate pain. Strengthening the abdominals is important for balancing muscles of the back.

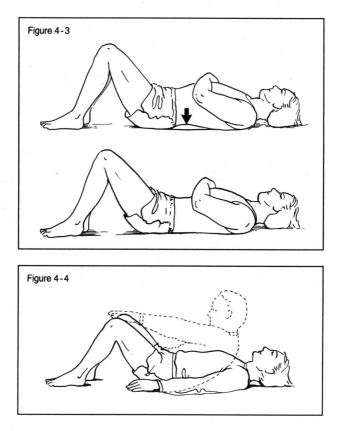

Figure 4-3

Figure 4-4

Elbow props and press-ups are particularly good for disk pain. Lying face down, the head and chest are raised off the floor, arching the low back until elbows can be used to prop up the chest. As pain diminishes and motion increases, the back arch progresses beyond elbow height to where the hands are actually used, pressing upward, accentuating the normal low back curve (Figure 4-5) and reducing the pressure on the disk. As usual,

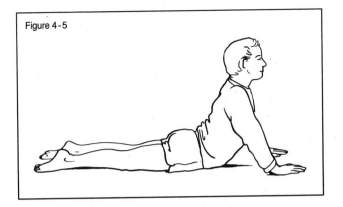

Figure 4-5

stretches should be held for 30 to 60 seconds to achieve maximal benefit. Ideally, these exercises should be routine in most people's lives for prevention but they can also help to waylay back pain once it has already started.

Other adjunctive treatments to help the hunter with back pain are heat, with either heating pad or hot shower and a use of thermal linaments with massage to loosen the muscles. These modalities are beneficial in reducing muscle pain and spasm. Using oral anti-inflammatory agents such as aspirin or Ibuprofen is usually quite effective for backache, whatever its cause. It may be taken four to six times a day without serious side effects. Gastritis, the most common side effect of these pills can be lessened by taking them immediately after eating a meal. I would not recommend the use of narcotics such as codeine or muscle relaxant prescriptions while hunting. They not only deaden the pain but also deter judgment. If you do have a prescription, they are only to be taken in the evening after hunting.

Positioning and support of the back are vital. Using a small pillow, a rolled-up towel or blanket and placing this in the low back arch while driving a car or sitting in any chair provides back support and helps maintain a more normal curve. Elastic lumbar corsets or braces can be worn beneath your hunting gear and provide relief by limiting motion as well as supporting the spine.

Warm-up the first thing in the morning, going through the aforementioned back therapy. This extra 10 minutes spent in the morning usually makes the remainder of the day more tolerable.

Limit your gear to essentials and pack it in smaller and lighter parcels. Use of a boat trailer or the lightest possible boat also saves one from very strenuous and clumsy lifting. It's often not necessarily the amount of weight but rather how it is lifted. Technique is important. Bend the knees, not the back and keep the load lifted close to the body.

When in the blind and your back starts hurting, move around, change positions, stand up and stretch, arching backwards for 30 seconds or even take a brief walk to move the joints. Arch your back frequently throughout the day, relieving the pressure on the lumbar disk. Change your position slowly so you don't alert ducks in the air and alienate your partner. If all else fails, brief chiropractic adjustment may at times help relieve the pain, particularly if your back has a painful catch in it from a sudden twist or a lift. These pinched facet syndromes cause pain that make someone stuck in the forward flexed position and can be usually relieved by one manipulation. Surgery for a ruptured disk is indicated when there is persistent or progressive pain, numbness or weakness in the legs. Fortunately most heal by themselves and only 10% require surgical excision.

Like the common cold, back pain will continue to plague most everyone, usually at the absolute worst time. From the duck blinds to deer stands those stationary hunts are at risk when the combination of high emotional tension, increased physical demands, the possibility of poor mechanics and posture come together on a hunt. Proper planning and a preventive back exercise program are the best guarantee against backache.

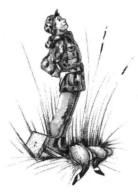

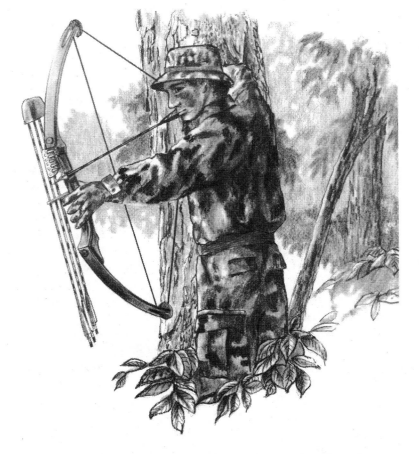

Chapter 5

Sportman's Shoulder
A Bowhunter's
Twang of Tendinitis

A t times he still could not believe it. For well over half of the
fifty-two years spent on this earth he had endured and
enjoyed a love affair with bow hunting and for the past five years,

had actually been paid to do so. Out from the cobwebs of the past he remembered his father's advice to find a job he could master and enjoy and hope that someone would pay him for it. Only a few months ago he had been hired to guide a few of the Minnesota Twins on a Wyoming mule deer hunt to be televised for an upcoming episode of the American Sportsman.

Often he recounted how it all began. He picked up his first bow while still in high school, an old but impressive recurve that belonged to his uncle. At that time Uncle Dave was considered eccentric by many of the local hunters for sneaking through the woods after local whitetails with a bow and arrow refusing to carry a traditional deer rifle. He was also well known as deadly accurate with the recurve from here to fifty yards. His uncle had taught him the proper technique of grip, pull, mount, hold, and release on paper plates nailed to a hay bale. Although he was impressed how accurate such a primative weapon could be it was the wood lore, the stalking and the tactical planning of bow hunting that enamored him to the sport. The entire process was different and somehow more intimate and personal than hunting with a rifle. Those were impressionable years and like all young men at that stage of life, he wanted to do it all and his major limitation seemed to be that each day had only twenty-four hours.

His autumn weekends were consumed by football games and weeknights with after school practices. Organized sports had been a major thrust in his life since he was old enough to throw a ball. But by his senior year, this new and exciting challenge of bow hunting had turned his head and it became a struggle to decide where to place his efforts when the leaves turned colors and fell to the ground. Gifted and energetic as he was, he maintained his high school athletics while still managing to occasionally steal away with his uncle to the quiet darkness of the hard woods and partially satiate his more primal desires. Some Saturdays would find him patiently on his stand for only a half an hour after day break. Then because of his prior committments, he raced home to participate in more "civilized" games.

For high school graduation, Uncle Dave bought him one of those new compound bows to take with him for companionship at the midwestern university he decided to call home for the next four years.

College seemed a whirl. Rapidly the months sped by with all the lectures, papers, parties, and ball games. A social young man, he made friends and many more acquaintances but each year when September played its beckoning, morning songs, he eagerly awaited the weekend to get out, alone, and away with his bow. Guns were not allowed on campus, but bows were a different story and he rarely returned empty handed. The patience and practice he allowed produced squirrels, rabbits, and an occasional grouse with blunt tip arrows and always provided a fat buck for his fraternity's fall banquet.

Luck and health remained with him. Despite all the organized sports that filled his early life he had never been injured. His string of luck ended however his junior year at the university. One October, Saturday afternoon while running a fly pattern for a long spiraling pass, the covering cornerback pushed him from behind at the most inopportune and unbalanced moment forcing him to jack-knife forward and fall with full momentum landing directly on his right shoulder. Minor sprain, the team Doc told him and in fact within two to three weeks, the incident was all but resolved except for a small lump and an occasional ache.

He had long forgotten the separated shoulder until now. Just one month away from the trip of a life time, not only being paid for something he'd rather do than breath, but he finally had made it to the big time, a chance on national television. He dreamt of future endorsements and a guide book that was filled two years in advance. His decision to maintain his proficiency with bow shooting, his central Wisconsin location he now called home, and of course his long time connection with college alumni had afforded him opportunities of which most could only dream. He took to the forest each fall guiding others who had only recently discovered the fulfillment of archery. His guided excursions were educational, with fast informational exchanges regarding edible local flora, weather signs, tracking, survival techniques and usually resulted in the harvest of a buck whitetail. He travelled to many other states, Alaska and even Canada in search of his game and eventually became a well known name around northern camp fires when the topic of bow hunting arose.

As an off season accountant, he had had a busy past year and was unable to practice much this summer. This, his third venture in the past two weeks to the straw bales confirmed his earlier fears that his shoulder hurt more each time he shot. Never before had he experienced similar pain. Well perhaps there was some aching at last season's end but not like this. It began to frighten and frustrate him. His grip and easy draw remained relatively strong, but when mounting to sight and holding a full draw shot, stabbing pains seared deep into his right shoulder. After ten or twelve arrows his strength faded making it difficult to initiate his draw at all. Over the next two weeks he experienced deep, toothache like pain in the shoulder at night, never severe enough to awaken him unless he tried to lie on that side. He had also noticed some loss of motion when he tried to lift his hand over his head or behind his back. He envisioned this trip passing before his eyes and with it his future as a professional bow hunting guide.

After much coaching and coaxing from his wife he visited his doctor and found out he was suffering from a "rotator cuff syndrome". He was relieved to know that this was not an arthritis that involved wearing out of the entire shoulder joint, but rather an inflammation localized to the shoulder cuff tendons (tendinitis) which coursed between the bony ball and socket. Also inflamed was the protective bursal sac (bursitis). Both of these structures had become so swollen and inflammed that it severely limited his motion. Thus faced with a significant loss of motion, a significant amount of pain, and considering the limited time before his trip, he elected to have a cortisone injection. The injection into his inflamed and swollen bursa took five minutes and within a week his shoulder had improved to the point that he could do the shoulder exercises the doctor prescribed and could even hold a full draw now. Not normal yet, but dramatically improved and target practice soon resumed.

Like most inflammatory conditions those involving the shoulder sneak up on you. They may be related to accumulative trauma from younger years, recently repeated strains and overuse or at times comes seemingly from nowhere and without cause.

The shoulder is a unique joint for two reasons. First, it is the most mobile joint of the body and this freedom of the ball within the socket can lead to excessive sliding and frictional wear to soft tissue structures around it. Secondly, it is the only joint with a muscle tendon actually that courses through a joint. This tendon is

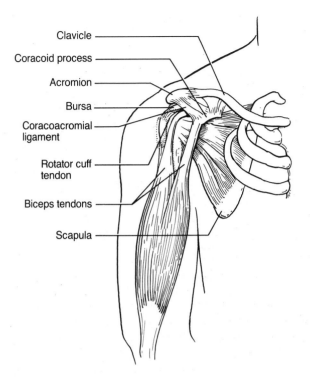

Clavicle
Coracoid process
Acromion
Bursa
Coracoacromial ligament
Rotator cuff tendon
Biceps tendons
Scapula

a broad, flat extension of four muscles that originate on the wing bone or scapula and insert on the humerus just below its ball and is called the rotator cuff. These muscles functioning through this thick tendon complex, elevate the arm to the side and rotate it inward and outward. Because of its location just beneath the roof of the shoulder and because of the inherent mobility possible the cuff is repeatedly compressed and rubbed as the ball pinches it against the roof. Over years of even normal shoulder use this vital cuff wears thin and becomes more susceptable to inflammation. With repeated inflammatory episodes or strains the cuff may weaken and even tear. It has been shown that men over sixty are likely to have at least small rotator cuff tears, regardless of their life's activity, but often times these minor tears produce few symptoms. This gradual process can be accelerated by overuse and

Bursa

Inflamed rotator cuff tendon

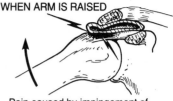

WHEN ARM IS RAISED

Pain caused by impingement of bursa and rotator cuff.

abuse of the joint and we are aware of even young throwing athletes that have been sidelined indefinitely by rotator cuff problems.

The shoulder bursa is a sac like structure whose primary responsibility is to protect the cuff from wear. This bursa rests like a deflated balloon lying between the rotator cuff and the bony roof of the joint. When the cuff is strained or inflammed special cells lining the bursa secrete fluid to fill the sac and provide a sort of water balloon type cushion for the cuff. When this occurs, the sac itself becomes thickened, swollen and is more likely to be pinched resulting in an even more fluid secretion and soon elevation of the arm above shoulder height causes repetitive impingement and a painful bursitis. The shoulder at this point loses significant motion especially reaching overhead or behind the back. Rotator cuff tendonitis syndrome is common particularly in the middle age, recreational athlete. The susceptability to it depends on the age and also the type of sport involved.

Although bow hunters and target archers are quite prone because of the strain placed on the cuff to draw and mount the bow, they by no means have a corner on the market. Shotgunners and wing shooters likewise can develop the nagging discomfort, weakness, and loss of motion after having completed a masterful weekend of swinging their shot guns into position for action. The common denominator is abducting (elevating to the side) the arm forcefully and repetitively above shoulder height, thereby impinging the cuff and bursa. This is not to be confused with "trap shooter's shoulder" which results from repeated contusions to the bones and muscles in the front of the shoulder. This bruising is related to the direct blows the shoulder takes from excessive kick or from a gun grip which is too loose when mounted.

Because of our anatomical evolution, we cannot entirely stop the wearing of the rotator cuff, but we can slow it down and conditioning is the key. It is important to stretch the shoulder muscles each day by doing arm circles or otherwise moving the shoulder through a full range. Light weight lifting three times a week will maintain the tone of all the shoulder muscles including the cuff. If you have access to a Universal gym, bench presses, latissimus pull downs, and rowing will benefit and free weights can be used for curls, flies, reverse flies, and side arm lifts. If you have a history of shoulder problems refrain from over head lifting as in military presses or pull overs. Push-ups are another excellent shoulder exercise that can be done at home. To selectively strengthen the cuff free weight side arm elevations (Figure 5-1) are initially used and then some form of a recoiling elastic resistance device such as surgical tubing or theraband is implemented to strengthen rotation itself.

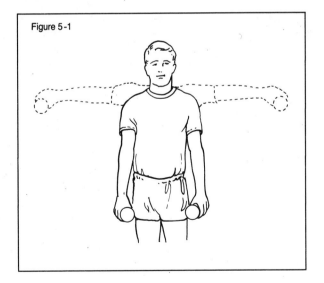

Figure 5-1

Four feet of surgical tubing can be purchased at most pharmacies, hospital supply houses or believe it or not in deep sea sports stores where it is used as artifical fish bait. The diameter varies with the tension desired and is wise to start with a size close to the diameter of your little finger. It can be purchased by the foot and is relatively inexpensive. Loops are tied at both ends of the four foot section of tubing one to hold in the hand and the other to hook on to a door knob or wall attachment. Rotational exercises are performed by turning sideways ninety degrees away from the door when one end of the tube is fixed to the door knob, with the tube clenched in one hand and the elbow remaining close to the waist (Figure 5-2). Internal rotation is performed twenty-five to fifty times and then the body is turned 180 degrees to face the opposite direction and external rotation is performed for a similar number of repetitions. This looks much like you are painting the wall with horizontal brush strokes with your elbow fixed at your side. After a few weeks when you have gradually achieved 100 repetitions of both internal and external rotations, the elbow can gradually be brought away from the waist to make more functional movements (Figure 5-3A & B). This is important because when hunting we rarely keep our elbows at our side, but rather have them elevated at least to some degree. Very rarely do we need to elevate our elbows above shoulder height however so it's not necessary to increase the risk of cuff impingement by working the tube overhead. More tension and therefore more resistance on the tubing can be provided by moving away from the door, thus stretching the tube requiring more work per repetition.

Tubing can also easily similate the bow hunters pull by facing the door knob attachment and pulling upward to the cheek and holding much as knocking an arrow. Be innovative and design your own functional program to meet your specific need, but remember to work out initially with the elbow positioned down at the side and go above shoulder height when the shoulder pain has completely gone. Perform multiple repetitions for endurance strengthening, usually three sets of 25 repetitions.

Other reminders to save the season for those who have a tendency to develop sore shoulders are: 1) be cautious or avoid excessive over head work such as painting ceilings, hanging windows, and so on, prior to the season, 2) start your shoulder

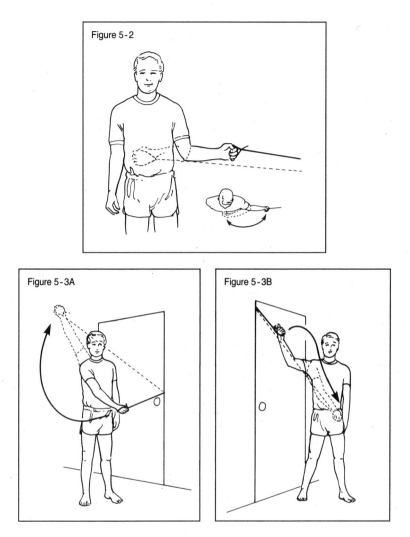

Figure 5-2

Figure 5-3A

Figure 5-3B

conditioning program four to six weeks prior to the season.

If pain develops during the course of the season, ice massage ten to twenty minutes three times a day, especially after exercise or activity and early use of anti-inflammatory agents such as aspirin or Ibuprofen may waylay a full blown syndrome. If the cuff syndome and shoulder pain progress, x-rays should be taken to see if calcium has formed in the shoulder. A judicious cortisone injection into the bursa usually gives dramatic relief in severe cases, but should not be repeated more than three times per year, for yearly repeated injections may actually weaken the cuff and predispose it to tearing more easily. In severe recurrent or chronic cases, surgical removal of the bursa and widening of the shoulder roof and if needed repair of a torn rotator cuff tendon usually serves the hunter well.

Whether the initial treatment of oral or injectable medication is successful or the tendinitis persists and requires surgery, the conditioning of the shoulder muscles is necessary to prevent recurrent shoulder pain. Well conditioned muscles absorb stressfull joint reaction forces and also stabilize the shoulder joint preventing the impingement phenomenon.

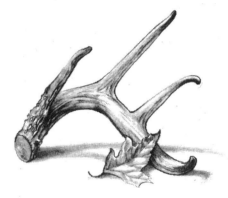

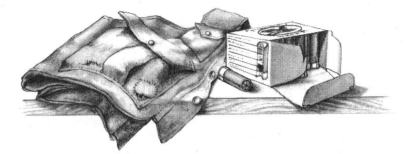

Chapter 6

Birdshooter's Forearm

I t was one of those rare years that swing by every so often that
make a person thankful to be alive, healthy, and able to share
the brilliance of a long Pennsylvania autumn. A record setting,
mild winter combined with a dry and abrupt spring provided the
proper setting for gallinaceous romance and subsequent ample
hatches of upland birds. There must be other explanations,
scientific or mythical and such theorizing brews long and well
over hot coffee and a fireplace loaded with blazing hickory logs.
But for the present, the bottom line was western Pennsylvania was
abundant with game birds. It was a year that could not be
explained simply by the peak cycle of ruffs whose booming filled
each vine clogged hollow. Ringnecks made an amazing advance
and strutted through alfalfa fields at an all time high. Even hardy
little plumps of bobwhite were scattered among the blackberries
that bordered many valley grain fields. Such an assortment with
such quantity made you glad to be a Pennsylvania bird hunter.

Daybreak found the brothers selectively stuffing shells into their
vests as they sat in a pickup sipping on strong black java. It had
become a new rite of each day's hunt this season watching the sun
come up, dunking powdered donuts and planning the morning's
movements. During this gray time of day boxes of shells emerged
from behind and under the seat; boxes marked high base, low

base, 4's, 6's and 8's in a rainbow of assorted colors. Most hunters, being the superstitious animals they are, savor the selection of their private collection of shells, usually of varying size, color and power. Somehow a patterned arrangement of these shells in the vest and in the shotgun magically bring more efficiency to the shooter and this season was a shot shellers dream. As the morning tactics were finalized and each different patch of cover reflected upon, a different box was brought up, passed, and a separate section of the vest isolated for a particular shell grouping.

They leave the truck as quietly as their boisterous labs allow, and slip through the partially harvested corn field looking for the roosters they spotted in this area in early September. Green #6's should be adequate, particularly lucky for some unknown reason this October morning but the trailing gunner skirting the edge of the field had better back up with a couple of red #4's. This frosty foray will deposit them down along the bottom land dotted with small stagnant ox-bow ponds thickly woven with alder, wild grape and nettles. At this junction, after drawing straws, they separate. The short straw wades the bend in the slow moving creek, the other two venture in wide arcs a mile along the river, one up and one down, only to return jump shooting in hopscotch fashion toward the center post man.

Along this bushy stretch of river they had hung over two dozen duck boxes through the years, dating back to when wood ducks were illegal game. The wood duck, beautiful to a fault, but also rigorous and prolific rose to the occasion and propagated to shootable numbers, no doubt thanks to the motley assortment of tree house condos made from plastic buckets, stovepipes, and wooden boxes. Very few animals sit more aware of their environment or fly a tree-dodging course so rapidly and gracefully as the woody. They take as much lead or steel as a ringneck but offer only snap shots and are hard to hit, much like partridge. In late season, a 6-4 or a 6-4-2 combination in the automatic would be just magic. A way back 2 is too powerful for jump shooting wood ducks or the occasional mallard, but was carried in reserve for luck with optimistic hopes that a few Canada's might have floated in to one of the hidden oxbows just around the bend.

After a bite of replenishment and another round of the shell game, it is off to the grapes and crabapples in search of thunder.

There has even been a change of shotguns, casing the automatics and pumps and now cradling light, open-bore doubles. As the sun rises high, the crispness remains and the crimson of maples and wide yellow pads of grape leaves provide a striking setting while the rotten sweetness of apples scattered on the ground lend aroma. Repeated bump and jump opportunities arise and even a bird or two fall for dinner. As the commercial goes "It just doesn't get any better than this". It is in a season such as this that you want nothing to distract you and nothing to go wrong.

As so often happens however, the better the hunting, the more you hunt and the more you hunt the more you become at risk of developing overuse syndromes of the muscles and joints. The most frequent presentation is a gradual onset of pain aggravated by activity, lingering through the evening. This subtle signal usually represents some form of an early tendinitis. Upland game hunters frequently develop overuse problems in the wrists, forearms, and elbows. The cause is related to carrying this gorgeously inlaid six to eight pound metal pipe around all day and using it in a variety of different positions and situations. It results from repetitive, rapid and forceful precision positioning of the shotgun as well as the less dramatic but also necessary toting the shotgun in a "ready" position.

Forearm syndromes are well known to all those who swing racquets for enjoyment on a tennis court or racquetball club and commonly is referred to as "tennis elbow". Now wait a minute, tennis elbow in a hunter? No connection is apparent between the two sports until you analyze the biomechanical muscle forces they share. One swings a 1 to 2 pound racquet with extreme force and the other swings a seven pound shotgun with similar force and precision.

In actuality forearm tendinitis often times is not related to the mount as much as to the carry. Those who have developed a habit of carrying their shotgun slung over their shoulder with one hand are constantly using their dominant upper extremity and eventually will notice after a few hours that their arm movement is slower. This can happen early in the day because of fatigue and later due to tired or aching, overused, forearm muscles. In hunters this overuse syndrome usually develops in the dominant arm.

Most muscles of the forearm are anatomically unique in that

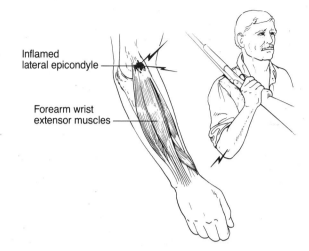

Inflamed lateral epicondyle

Forearm wrist extensor muscles

they cross at least two joints. The majority start just above the elbow and insert into bones of the hand as they cross the wrist. Their function is to move the elbow, wrist and fingers in flexion, extension and rotation. Other unique characteristics of these muscles are that they must provide extremely powerful actions while at the same time be precisely coordinated. This double duty of forcefulness in carrying a gun and reacting to a flush and precision when mounting, releasing the safety and pulling the trigger all in an instant may result in tendinitis if your mechanics are faulty or if you arm muscles are out of shape and not prepared for the task at hand.

The typical aching feeling is usually located around the elbow, but at times can radiate into the forearm and even into the wrist. It feels like a deep toothache in the elbow and often times it is sore to touch, more so on the lateral prominence or epicondyle of the elbow where the muscles insert into bone. There is very little swelling or discoloration of the skin at this point. The pain definitely becomes worse with any resisted motion while lifting even a light load such as coffee pot and rotating the forearm while opening a door. Whatever you call it; elbow tendinitis, epicondylitis, tennis elbow, birdshooter's forearm can be nagging and definitely ruin your entire season.

If you are a bird shooter, your preseason conditioning program should include forearm exercises to strengthen these muscle groups. Five to ten pound dumbbells can be used for wrist curls and extensions in three to four sets of 10 repetitions. These are done while sitting with your forearm lying along the top of a table or bench. Using your opposite hand to hold and support the wrist, the dumbbell is lowered and raised much like an elbow curl except the movement occurs only at the wrist. The forearm is then turned over so that the palm faces down and three to four sets of 10 repetitions are repeated for wrist extension (Figure 6-1). The wrist extension exercise is most important to prevent forearm tendinitis. Rotation strength can be improved by sitting in a similar position holding the hammer, the head pointed toward the ceiling, then rotating it side to side multiple times. Additionally elbow curls and hand grip strengthening are beneficial.

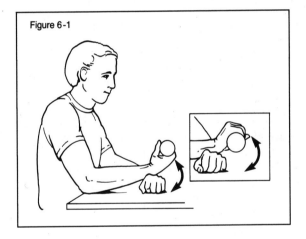

Figure 6-1

This forearm overuse syndrome is not merely a question of muscle strength or weakness but includes other factors including the weight and balance of the shotgun, the number of times it's lifted, the position from where the gun is mounted, the speed and force of each mount. Therefore if forearm/elbow pain develops during the season, a number of practical activity modifications may be necessary. It is obvious that a poorly balanced and cheaply made double side by side that is butt heavy requires more work than a sleek six pounder with balance. Theoretically the

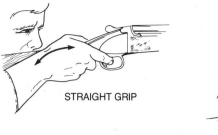

STRAIGHT GRIP

PISTOL GRIP

European straight grip forces the wrist into more flexion and may put the forearm muscles at a disadvantage. I am not suggesting we burn our English stocks, but those who have recurrent bouts of elbow tendinitis may want to try more vertical pistol grip stock.

For hunters who have had forearm tendinitis in the past it makes sense to plan your day's hunt where a lighter gun can be carried in the afternoon, perhaps even switching from a 12 gauge to a 20 if you have one available and shed a pound or two. If all your shotguns are twelves, this condition provides one of the all time truthful and irrefutable albeit medical excuses for purchasing that slim, smooth, 5½ pound 20 gauge that you have been dreaming about for years. Afterall, what is a forearm worth if it's so painful that it can't hug a spouse or snap up on a pheasant threading its way skyward through a tule swamp. If presented to the wife with the arm wrapped in a bandage, a bottle of Napa Valley Chardonnay and some pain in your voice, at times this medical prescription tactic even works.

If you are able to switch gauges in the same day, be safe and certain to carry an extra vest. This is the ultimate shell game played with two different vests, two different gauges and a variety of new colors, sizes and perhaps even different heavy metals. The risk of slipping a 20 gauge shell into your 12 gauge is obviously much greater than developing any overuse syndrome, therefore if guns and gauges are switched, be certain that all shells are likewise, hence the wisdom of a 20 and a 12 gauge vest.

Think for a minute how you usually carry your shotgun — everyone has their favorite position. As previous researchers and authors have pointed out, the shotgun carry is most efficient at port arms. It gets the gun on the game quicker. It also effectively prevents repeated abuse of your dominant arm by spreading the load over both forearms and utilizing all muscle groups in both arms. Much like swinging the golf club, carrying the gun in front with both hands allows the lead nondominant hand to absorb most of the force, leaving the dominant one free for precision positioning. Keep the shotgun close to the body, not way out front. Just this simple change dramatically reduces the work of shoulder and arm muscles by effectively shortening the mechanical lever arm and thus the force necessary to raise the gun. For the bird hunter the shotgun stays lighter longer and hopefully more accurate.

If the familiar ache has already settled in and the season is still young, treatment for the tendinitis may salvage the remainder of the year. Stretching the stiff muscles is done by extending the arm and elbow out straight with palm down, the wrist flexed and the back of the hand against the wall. Passively the back of the hand is then pushed against the wall and held for 30 to 60 seconds, stretching the muscles on the top of the forearm and elbow (Figure 6-2). Stretching exercises should be performed for two to three minutes, three to four times a day and at least once a day they should be followed by previously outlined weight lifting program of wrist and elbow curls and extensions.

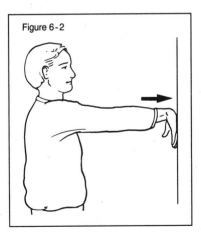

Figure 6-2

Icing directly on the sore spot along the forearm and about the elbow for 10 minutes three to for times a day is likewise helpful in reducing the inflammation. Finally, using a prefabricated tennis elbow band or sleeve at times provides amazing relief. These elastic or neoprene bands can be bought at most athletic supply stores. How and for whom they work is still a mystery but they are easy to apply and adjust, and definitely provide supportive compression around the forearm muscles.

The combination of a 20 gauge double, a uniform of nylon faced brush busters and a neoprene elbow band would be enough to cause rumblings from the graves of the past masters of bird shooting, but when the season is hot and the birds are flocked and flushing, anything goes and there is no right or wrong way to enjoy the wings of autumn.

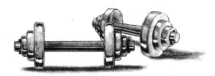

Chapter 7

Imaging
Honing the Psychological Edge

In sports arenas so competitive that mere milliseconds separate the winners and losers, it comes down to more than pure physical effort. The outcome is often determined by the mental and emotional edge. We hear it every year at playoff time; the winner will be the one with desire, focus and superior psychological edge.

Have you ever wondered how Larry Bird sinks 90% of his free throws, Ted Williams batted consistently for a .350 average, or Edwin Moses continued to smoke over high hurdles past his opponents in record time? These elite athletes share one common characteristic that makes them superstars. They recognize and practice the art of imaging. Sports psychologists have developed this concept of imaging by observing and questioning the mental patterns and practices of successful athletes. How a team or an individual achieve their goal remains a combination of many complex factors but in the psycho sports world, imaging has become a method to gain the edge, to polish and peak a performance.

The concept is an old one, practiced in many fields of endeavor, often times unknowingly. Competitive trap shooters, the ones that consistently break 100 out of 100 are stars at this game. Ask enough of them just what their secret of success is and answers like; heredity, hard work, practice ethics and skill will be bounced around. Under closer scrutiny all will relate mental practice periods of 100% concentration, mentally visualizing the entire event, act by act. Imaging trains them to concentrate and focus with intensity on the clay pigeon, it's probable speed and angle of flight, blocking out all else and so doing the event is carried out smoothly and efficiently.

On the range or in the woods, voluntary or not, imaging can give an amazing boost to your confidence as a shooter. Concentration is the name of the game. Agreed, but how can someone practice concentration? Imaging is taught to athletes through a number of techniques. Some sports psychologists replay video tapes reviewing the proper technique until over time it becomes imprinted in the person's mind. The player then spends time before games in brief but intense concentration remembering the image of the technique and then projecting himself into this visualization and into the present tense.

Most of us use to play the image game as kids. As a 14 year old junior member of the Boston Celtics, game on the line, he imagines himself at the foul line, no time left on the clock, one point behind and a chance at a 1 on 1. His mind is fixed, he sees each step run rapidly through his mind; the foot placement, three dribbles, the feel of the ball, the roar of the crowd, concentrating, concentrating on the front rim of the basket, the shot, arc, and follow-through all the way to the point of seeing the ball go through the hoop. As you can see, the shot itself is the goal but still a very small part of the entire process. Practicing the mental steps definitely will improve shot percentage, be it basketballs or bluebills.

You may presently be practicing your own type of imaging without knowing it. Certainly deer hunters often season themselves against the heartbreak of buck fever, by closing their eyes and imagining sights, sounds, and feelings of an approaching ten point buck, how he would stand, the aim, and finally the hit. At first glance it may seem that imaging is suited only for the big game hunter where the game is sighted afar. There is time for an approach, either the game to you or you to it, followed by subsequent aiming and shooting process. This scenario does not present itself often throughout a season so there is much time to practice.

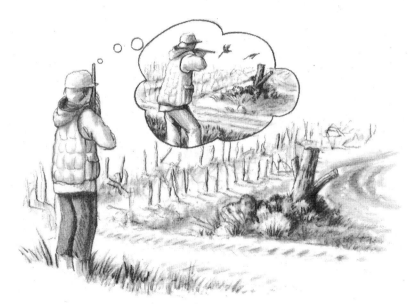

Bird hunters can likewise benefit from imaging. Each time they approach a likely looking cover they should anticipate their approach based on the bird's most likely route of escape. Quickly and thoroughly inspect the cover the bird must fly through, looking for the tunnels in the trees or foilage openings that provide the avenues of flight. All attention should then be placed on the cover and all senses, particularly sight and sound are directed with intensity toward that suspicious looking thicket that might be hiding a bird. With the first rustling of leaves or beat of wings as the bird jumps, your gun is already at port and your intensity will be focused. If the bird selects one of the tunnels that you have already imaged, such as; splitting the two pine trees, skimming the edge of the corn field or ducking in and out of the fire lane, locating, tracking with the shotgun and placing your charge will likely meet with a bird belly-up on the forest floor.

In time the pattern becomes second nature. Some might label it intuition, some call it luck, but in the final analysis it is the process practiced by all successful hunters. I have always thought of hunting as at least one-half anticipation and the other half eye/hand coordination beautifully blended with a healthy dose of aerobic physical effort. That is certainly not to say that game is predictable and that they will always pick the same holes in the wall of woods that you do, but that's what makes us love the sport and keeps us coming back.

During a day, everyone at some point loses their mental concentration as their mind drifts to unconscious daydreaming. At times in such a situation a surprise flush will be dropped with a rapid and skillfully placed snap shot. It is fun to be lucky, isn't it? However, you are much more likely to find something in your game bag at the end of the day by anticipating and imaging your shot before the bird flushes than by wandering the woods with a rabbit's foot, and a snap shot. Stalking fields and forests haphazardly just hoping to scare up game may do just that but very rarely offers a good chance for a shot.

It is always difficult to image prior to hunting a new area. You are unfamiliar with the cover, the unique actions and responses of local game, it may be raining, and hundreds of other variables make it impossible the first day out. So the initial day or so spent in a new area should be approached with a somewhat laid-back, exploring type attitude and as the familiarity grows, so does the ability to anticipate. The ability to "read cover" usually determines how rapidly this acclimatization occurs. Once you are familiar with the cover that you are to hunt, spend 5 to 10 minutes the night before and again the morning of the hunt in quiet solitude, imagining; where your partner, your dog, and you will be walking, the pace, the stops at likely looking thickets, also remembering where previous birds have flown on prior trips through this area.

One can almost think of imaging as a very brief but intense meditation on a particular action or maneuver, how you perceive it will occur and how you will accomplish your goal. Wild idea? No, most of us image frequently to some degree for it encourages focusing one's attention, blocks out any distractions and gives you the edge on your game. Remember hunting is a head game.

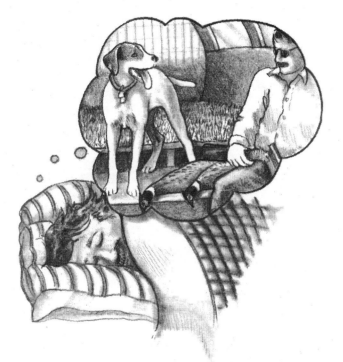

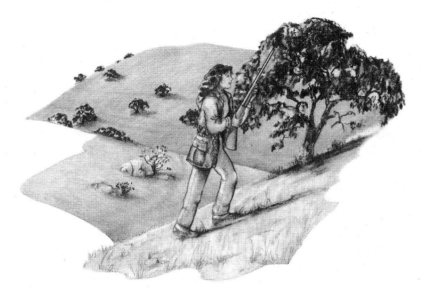

Chapter 8

Hill Tops and Knee Caps

I f you'd ask, most would simply answer that she beat to a different drummer, and that she always had. Twenty-five years ago she was born the sole offspring and heir to a fortunate pair, both of whom had a strong love for outdoor adventure. Even during her first year of life she often could be found tailgate riding behind her mother as they biked along country roads or bouncing by high atop her father's shoulders nestled in his backpack. By age five she had become an avid fan of fishing anywhere, anyway, and by eight, she could wield her father's seven foot graphite fly rod with astonishing accuracy. In her early years, her dad also taught her the art of plinking tin cans with a twenty-two, hitting bails of oat straw with arrows shot from her miniature twenty pound recurve and eventually, shooting clay pigeons with a twenty-eight gauge Remington 1100 that he just happened to suspiciously pick up in a fire sale one year.

As a family, their annual vacations involved hiking and camping to rugged, far-away places and so developed her keen appreciation for nature. Her mother usually participated and always encouraged these outdoor activities thought by some to be quite "unladylike". But her parents had always thought of her first as a person, not as a girl.

Fortunately she grew up at a time of social evolution when girls were categorized neither as china dolls nor tomboys. In fact, tomboy was a term that seemed to be rapidly phasing out as the baby boomer generation grew into parenthood. The boomers' children seemed to feel less pressure from their parents and their peers to be locked into gender roles and it was just as acceptable for a boy to be a musician and get A's on his report card as it was for a girl to be athletic and student council president. Thus she grew up, as psychologists would offer, well adjusted and more importantly blessed with a rare blend of knowledge and talent.

But something happened. As it often does during that confusing, corruptable, unsettling time of life known as adolescense. Many of her close friends changed and new roles evolved so that by time college rolled around, new thoughts as to how young ladies should be swept through the ranks of peers and parents. It somehow seemed less acceptable to be an athletic outdoors woman. The species was becoming endangered.

Her cum laude years at the university had been replete as cheerleader, captain of the trap team, and even a sophomore stint as class president. She was very much an integral part of campus life, however, semester breaks and vacations found her anxious to arrive home, throw on some drab, well worn, cotton clothes and hiking boots and dive back to woods or streams with her parents, friends, or even alone. It was at this time in her life that she refined and polished all of her outdoor experiences and observations to the point her father claimed she was now more adept in the woods than he. Because of her incessant curiosity she studied nature's offerings and felt quite comfortable walking a deer path pointing out trees, fungi, vines, and anything green, naming each and reciting its niche for human or wildlife consumption, shelter, or even medicinal uses. Similarly she could stalk a whitetail, hit a grouse on the wing and blow a mean mallard come back call from the confines of her duck blind.

She felt very secure with her life, but also acutely aware that others at times felt very uneasy with her presence. She remembered the faces on the good old boys at the skeet range and how their jaws dropped when they first witnessed her break twenty-five straight with her little twenty-eight gauge, the hesitancy of her father's hunting partners when he told them he was bringing his daughter on the trip and the prideful surprise felt by all when her chocolate lab, Bruno, came in second in the state hunter-simulated retriever trials. She would raise eyebrows, standing in line for an early morning duck blind pick at the state refuge. She was amused by the reaction of the bearded, low talking, camoflauged men when the light inside the refuge quonset flashed on and she was the only female in this sea of men. They reacted not so much that a woman would be out there at five a.m. vying for a drizzling duck blind but that the woman would be attractive as well. She knew these feelings, had adjusted well, and could inauspiciously put them down to rest once those around her realized that she was for real. She ventured there in the rain and snow for all of the same reasons and with at least as much enthusiasm.

Although an ardent fan of many outdoor endeavors, it was hard to say what she enjoyed most. However she always found the excitement and solitude of upland birds a thrilling yet peaceful experience which provided a sense of serenity. Like upland gunning, her life in general had come together with persistence and much hard work and the efforts spent were worth the goals achieved. Her career as an innovative co-ed physical education teacher at the local high school was satisfying and although her family was under way, she still found time to retreat from the rat race and enjoy the simple pleasures. Now the problem was time. Time for participating in her many activities, and time that she felt was necessary for preparation. She felt particularly perplexed since the birth of her son eithteen months ago and how difficult it was to work her body back into shape. It seemed the more she tried, the more she was distracted by higher priorities and soon she would pay the consequence.

For two months the aggravating discomfort had persisted. Since returning from the long awaited chukar hunt along Oregon's

Klammath River ridges, she had noticed a nagging ache deep within her knees. It reminded her of a similar episode she experienced during the first month of volleyball practice at the university, but those pains gradually subsided within a few weeks while she worked out in the trainer's room after practice. From time to time since she would feel something in her knees, perhaps a snapping catch, perhaps an aching pain, but had always shrugged it off. In Oregon, however, there was no time to shrug it off.

She and her husband had spent a full six months collecting information about Northwestern chukars, had finally decided on the Klammath River area because of its notarity and vastness. They ultimately located a rancher in that area who gladly offered to serve as chauffer and guide on this, their first trip alone since the baby was born.

The seven hour plane ride provided a harbinger of things to come for by the time they landed, there was already a dull, cramping feeling beneath the knee caps made somewhat worse by a two hour, backseat, jeep ride to their ranch house accommodations. During the entire trip, she never did adjust to those bumpy, dusty rides in the back of the jeep with no leg room. Then there were the hills, all the hills, nothing tremendously steep, but all unforgivingly ascended and descended for what seemed an eternity until after three days of up and down, she longed for one long flat stretch. But the weather was glorious this time of year and the rolling hills and steep creek cut banks that went on forever intrigued her with those natural elements plus an abundance of red legged, v-throated, silver feathered rockets of white meat and her intense desire to follow their new Lewellyn setter she was able to turn off outside irritations temporarily and went on to experience what she considered to be one of her "dream hunts."

Each evening however, she felt gimpy after arising from dinner, but a couple of aspirin and a short walk down the ranch road and the stiffness seemed to subside. It was not until the plane trip home that she really appreciated the pain, not sharp and stabbing, but more like a deep ache right behind the knee cap, a cramping sensation that made her want to move the knees back and forth or at least straighten them out for a while. This was the first time that she also noticed a definite swelling around her knees as well.

In typical "get busy and I'll get better" attitude, she tried as best she could to rest her legs after returning, but when a rare, free weekend came, her twenty-eight gauge called to her from the gun cabinet, and she could not resist. From then on, each time out was a struggle until finally her longest hunting season came to a close.

That last Saturday evening as she sat on the couch singing softly to her son, her mind drifted and imagined just what it would be like for the professional ball player who had been lucky enough to stay healthy and remain free of medical problems for eight years in the bigs, only then to suffer his first injury. At first there is denial and frustration then thoughts of aging and finally as the pain persists, a vague sense of fear as to its cause and cure. All athletes reach this point some time in their career. For most, the knee joint is the weak link in the musculoskeletal chain. "It's the knees that go first" it's been said through the years. Contusions, tortional sprains, and a variety of painful inflammatory conditions occur with rather alarming frequency and well over half are specifically related to the knee cap or patella.

The patella develops within the quadriceps tendon and acts as a moving fulcrum through which the quadriceps can exert its force to extend the knee. Its presence increases the quardriceps power at least four fold. Superficially the patella feels like a circular disk of bone, but the opposite, joint-side forms a triangular wedge that courses along a groove in the femur bone. Each time the knee moves, the patella tracks along this groove, but not always in a perfect line. Often times being tethered laterally by tight ligaments it courses just off center. When this common anatomical variant is present an abnormal wear pattern to the joint cartilage may occur as most of the pressure is being applied to only the outside surface of the patellar triangle. The cartilagenous surfaces of the patella are the thickest in the body, often a quarter inch or more, belying the fact that this joint accepts and usually tolerates tremendous force from pressure and friction. With continued repetitive high torque force on this joint it is not surprising that it frequently presents as a source of pain.

Our understanding about knee cap pain is far from complete, but certain aspects have been well defined. There are certain individuals prone to develop patellar pain syndromes. Those are individuals with loose or dislocating knee caps, abnormal leg alignments such as in-toeing or out-toeing, legs with relative

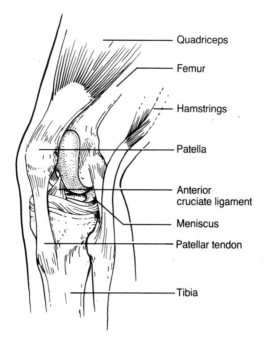

Quadriceps

Femur

Hamstrings

Patella

Anterior
cruciate ligament

Meniscus

Patellar tendon

Tibia

weakness in their quadricep for whatever reason, and also patellae that have absorbed direct trauma such as from a dashboard during an automobile accident or a fall directly on the knees. Patellar pain is notoriously more frequent in women than men perhaps due mainly to a greater degree of knock knees inherent in women as a result of a slightly broader pelvis. By no means, however, is this exclusively a female condition. The weekend warrior male or female, who lives a rather sedate, nonphysical existence five days a week and then come Saturday, attempts rapid transformation into a physical animal even with gardening, house maintenance, or especially with strenuous sports activities eventually will experience this discomfort.

Activities that stress and pressure the knee cap such as kneeling, squatting, ascending and descending stairs or hills and forceful running and jumping are those guaranteed to produce pain. The discomfort to some degree comes from repetitive strain of the quadricep muscles that tries to control the patella's course in the femoral groove, but also from inflammation of the cartilage

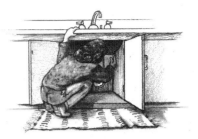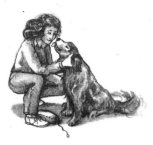

surface itself. Except for kneeling, (direct pressure) all the activities that aggravate the patella demand strong quadricep muscles and simply put, "so goes the quad, so goes the patella." Like an automobile shock spring system protects the tires, if the quadricep is weak and cannot provide the shock absorption, all forces are directed to the knee cap which, after a time, responds by becoming inflamed and sore. Over years of abuse the patellar cartilage can become soft, worn, and develops into what medical personnel call chondromalacia the literal translation of which is "bad cartilage."

This is not to say that normal use and wear is without some change. As you recall the first time you noticed a sensation of grinding or grating in your knee and the surprise and perhaps shock that grabbed you. Getting old? Wearing out? Or is this an old injury returning to haunt you? In actuality it may be a little of each. This clicking noise is normal, for nearly everyone over twenty-five years of age will have undergone some wear of the cartilage, some softening and ridging and experience occasional grinding noise that represents a washboarding effect as two joint surfaces glide over one another. In the normal knee this grinding-grating sensation is usually not painful and by itself is no cause for alarm or concern about arthritis. In some cases, however, the quadriceps and patellae are pushed well beyond their capabilities and it is then that chondromalacia becomes symptomatic and of concern.

At that point the individual may notice a slight limp and in bilateral conditions, the legs may feel weak and rubbery even after typical daily activities. Sitting for a prolonged time and with knees bent such as at a theater or on a long auto trip, will create stiffness and a feeling that the joint needs to be "oiled." In people who have a proponderance for this condition, heavy knee demand such as hunting hills may create acute flares of chondromalacia which may even be associated with swelling and fluid in the knee, a certain sign of marked inflammation.

As usual, in prevention and treatment, there are some things we can change and some we cannot. If the patella recurrently dislocates or jumps out of place, a surgical correction affords lasting results. The surgery is performed arthroscopically and directed at releasing the tight lateral ligaments that hold the patella to the side.

If you are one of many in-toers or quite the opposite and walk like a duck, an orthotic arch support can provide a neutral foot base thereby preventing the rotational torque on the knee cap. Specially prescribed knee sleeves and straps at times can benefit those with acute and even chronic symptoms. These sleeves are fashioned from neoprene or elastic and usually provide a pad that pushes laterally on the patella and helps keep it tracking properly in the groove.

Patellar pain of any etiology, particularly if related to intense weekend or seasonal activity, responds well to quadricep strengthening. Strong quadriceps stabilize hypermobile knee caps and also readily absorb the stresses of excessive walking, running or climbing. Conditioning should first start with three to five minutes of flexibility warm-ups stretching both the quadriceps and hamstrings (Figure 8-1A & B). Then sitting at a high chair or counter, free weights such as velcro ankle weights or simply a purse or knapsack filled with a predetermined weight are hung over the ankle. Bent knee exercises are performed gradually extending the knee fully and holding for a five second count, then gradually lowering the weight back toward the floor until ninety degrees flexion at the knee is reached (Figure 8-2). The amount of weight used depends on the symptoms and reason for the exercise. In a preseason conditioning program, one can start with ten pounds and increase the weight weekly by ten pounds with a limit of approximately thirty to fifty pounds, depending on the size, sex and age of the individual. If the person is recovering or rehabilitating from a painful flare-up of knee pain, they should start with five pounds and increase in five pound increments. Multiple repetitions (3 to 5 sets of 10 repetitions) maximize knee

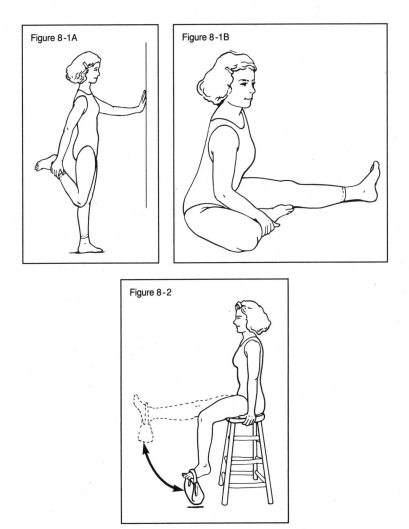

Figure 8-1A

Figure 8-1B

Figure 8-2

cap and quadricep endurance. It is much more important to do three sets of twenty repetitions with twenty pounds than it is to do five repetitions with one hundred pounds per leg.

Other exercises that benefit the quadricep are wall squats, leg presses on a weight machine, bicycling, and working out on cross country ski or rowing machines. The recently developed stair stepper training devices fantastically simulate hill climbing and also provide low impact exercise for the leg. It is important again to remember the S.A.I.D. (Specific Adaptations for Imposed Demands) principle here and graduate slowly and progressively to walking, rope jumping, then jogging and finally climbing which more closely similates hunting activity. It should be obvious that a preseason conditioning program is the best preventive assurance.

One final item relates to medication. Compounds such as aspirin and Ibuprofen are very effective against patellar inflammation and can be taken in a dose of eight to twelve per day if symptoms persist. Usually after three to five days the aspirin compounds can be tapered and discontinued. The medicine will get you over the pain but it's the muscle conditioning that is necessary in the long run. Knee cap pain is an elusive, but very common and real source of discomfort and disability. Its appearance may wax and wane for years and to some degree one must learn to live with occasional aches, but through proper planning and conditioning this painful condition can be lessened or prevented altogether.

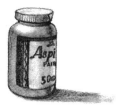

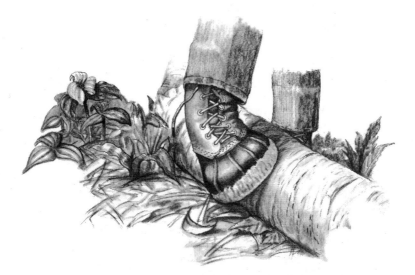

Chapter 9

Slippery Leaves and Ankle Sprains

L ike the low lying fog filling the valley, that unfounded feeling began to creep across the hackles of my neck. It was always like that when we hiked or hunted Whiskey Town Hollow, an eerie excitement that beckons with one whisper and cautions with another. If it were not for the bountiful supply of rust-red, ruffed grouse, I would turn around and sneak out. Not one to believe in the supernatural, I do however admit to just a touch of superstition and contend that when hunting this valley I feel a pressure to perform well almost as if eyes of the past remain watchfully passing judgment.

The hollow's history is as colorful as an October day as told by a few remaining octogenarians that live contentedly in wood frame shanties tucked away at the mouth of the valley. In the sixties, the Civil War sixties, it was a site of a Union foundry that casted pig iron into cannon balls, artillary shells and bayonet blades. At first glance, it looked like any other hollow in the lower Appalachian chain but early settlers came to realize that Mother Nature bestowed a unique combination of limestone and coal buried superficially in the surrounding hills and raw iron ore that lay along the bed of Whiskey Run. Sunken kilns were dug along the creek bank, lined with brick, filled with a combination of limestone, coal and iron ore and fired hot enough to chemically and mysteriously combine them. The molten pig iron then sank down to the kiln's bottom and flowed out a funnel like chute into the cannon ball and bayonet casts, which were then cooled by the hissing and steaming creek water. Horse drawn wagons bumped and swayed along the winding trail down to the kiln and then back again loaded with hardware for the Union army depot a hundred and twenty miles away. Suddenly the war ended and with it so died the demand for artillary shells. The foundry closed leaving many unskilled workers without income. Most eventually left in search of work in a more prosperous land.

Then left to their own devices, the surrounding hardwood floors of beech, oak, and hickory which had been harvested to fire the furnaces, regenerated. Early in this natural plant succession the local ruffed grouse population flourished and many felt the blasts of market gunners and found their way to the city, a repast for the wealthy. Old timers parlayed tales of phenomenal grouse harvests that grew exponentially each year as long as the trees were small and the forests somewhat open. But this golden era gradually faded as the heavy hardwood canopy occluded the sunlight so vital for underbrush growth. So goes the ground cover; so go the grouse. This ecological concept was not recognized by the market hunters and in their typical, imaginative manner explained the grouse away by either them "taking sick with plague", or more commonly "migrating to another area" hundreds of miles away.

Sometime later after the turn of the century, the Hollow's history was painted yet another color during those often dark, unpredictable years of prohibition. Where once there had been iron kilns, now there were whiskey stills. The narrow dirt lane that hugged the bank of Whiskey Run again saw the horse and wagon and even an occasional canvas covered truck transporting local grains in, and illegal mash liquor back out by cover of starlight. Once again the forests suffered. Some hardwood logs fired the stills while yet others burned very slowly in huge mounds (smothered with wet tarps) and under low oxygen conditions to form charcoal which was used to filter the whiskey and stabilize its taste. If not deliciously smooth, the final product was at least powerful and quite acceptable to the lower Appalachian gentry. The distillery flourished until word mysteriously leaked to the Feds.

The local constabulary low-profiled it, wanting no part in destroying the area's prime industry. But despite vocal warnings , the musty smell of fermenting grain wafted from the valley.

The inevitable showdown came just before dawn, one frosty November day in 1921 with the crack of a rifle and shouts from government agents as they rushed in to destroy stills and arrest bootleggers. Much to their dismal surprise, the hollow boys were not to be intimidated and the cat and mouse skirmish that continued intermittently over three days left nineteen good men dead for what both felt was just cause. Realizing they were out of their element, the G-men retreated but returned with reinforcements only to find the stills had been neatly disassembled and transported deeper into the forest to another and then another unnamed hollow. Thus the quaint little cluster of shanties known as Whiskey Town, disassembled and its citizens disappeared.

Ivy and creeper vines smothered the limestone foundations. Moss and ferns covered the rotting cords of hickory and oak saplings sprung from any open land as once again botanical succession hurried in to fill the void, doing so just in time to peak before the outlawing of market hunting. Slow to change, a few local gunners kept at their trade often taking hundreds of birds each month and selling them on the sly for a dollar a brace. They figured as long as the city market demand remained high and there were birds enough to fill it that certainly no one was about to enforce this assinine law. Grouse were thought to be in endless supply and they saw no reason to conserve.

Enforcement did indeed arrive sometime in 1934 in the form of a hard-nosed, stick to the rulebook warden and many are the tales of wild chase and escape through the upland and soggy bottoms of Whiskey Hollow.

Inevitably with such a rich cast of characters come the ghosts, not apparitions or haunts but rather deja vu feelings of early iron workers, saavy bootleggers and crafty market hunters, all gone but leaving skeletons of past endeavors and of course grouse to mark the spot. The whiskey town line of grouse, though never in numbers they once knew, still remain the largest and smartest in the state. Bagging such a bird in this valley reaches toward an almost mythical experience. So today like the fog that often lingers along the valley floor a strange sensation comes creeping like the cold dampness following an autumn thunder shower and with it, the feeling that something just might go wrong.

The day drew ashen, dreary and damp. Last night's storm left the forest floor littered with layers of wet, slippery, burnt orange oak leaves. Transversing a sidehill upward toward a clump of grapevine thicket, my companion's mind was riveted on the tangle, expecting the sudden thundering flush of the ruffed grouse that he just knew was there. The approach seemed simple as his entire body fixed on the suspicious clump of cover. With gun at port, he slowed his gait, listening for that first rustle of leaves. Without warning and as rapidly as a blast from his 12 gauge, his feet left the ground and he twisted and slipped to the turf in a heap, covered with the dampened, dead leaves.

The pain was immediate and perhaps there was a single snap at the ankle. He couldn't say because everything happened so fast. Feeling every bit ridiculous, he arose to inspect the culprit, a bark stripped oak log, many years fallen and lying in a vertical downhill fashion, hidden beneath the forest floor blanket. This antique snare, wet with rain and greased even further with leaves had innocently but most effectively interrupted the chase. Needless to say the pair of grouse that lurked in the grapevine no doubt chuckled a bit as they drummed away from their unfortunate morning visitors. He arose slowly, humbled, hurt and cursing his clumsiness.

"What happened?"

"Slipped!"

"Are you okay?"

"Yeah, I think so," shaking away the stars.

Falling while hunting was routine and something to take in stride but as the day progressed his boot felt tighter and ankle seemed stiffer and he could no longer tolerate the ups and downs, let alone walking the sidehills. A day made bleak and certainly not the way to start a three day week-end of partridge shooting in the Southern Appalachians. Back home, removing the rubber packs was not terribly painful but it was surprising how swollen and discolored the foot and ankle were so soon after the injury.

So it goes with the all too common lateral ankle sprain. This type of injury accounts for 25% of all time that is lost in competitive sports. But the high performance athlete does not monopolize the market for this injury. Countless hunting trips have been agonized over or cancelled altogether because of twisting the ankle just a bit too far. This usually occurs while walking or running through slippery or uneven terrain, perhaps marked with hidden obstacles such as fallen trees or stumps, roots or rocks. The foot turns inward and downward, very forcefully stretching and in some cases tearing the ligaments on the outside portion of the ankle. The ligaments, thus stretched beyond the point of elastic recoil, bleed with swelling and discoloration occurring subsequently.

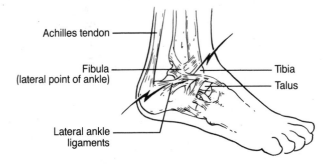

Prevention of ankle sprains is especially important for those with a history of prior sprains and those who have "loose ankles". Strengthening calf muscles with toe raises or performing isometric exercises at the ankle in four directions, up and down and side to side, applying force against an immoveable object and holding for five seconds is beneficial. Rubber surgical tubing the size of the diameter of your small finger can be purchased at most pharmacies in three to four foot lengths. A loop of the surgical tubing is tied around the forefoot and the four direction ankle exercises are repeated actively with motion, now resistance provided by the surgical tubing (Figure 9-1). Numerous repetitions, (50 to 100) in each direction are necessary for strengthening. Better balance and agility can be derived by rope jumping, box hopping or running drills such as carioccas.

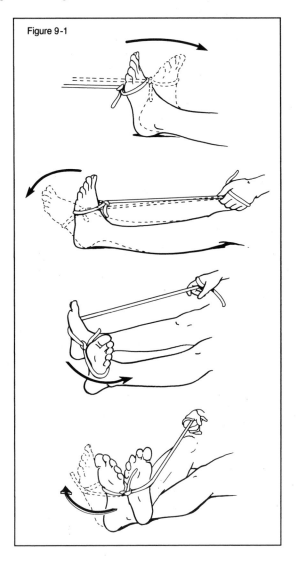

Figure 9-1

Boots with strong lateral supports that are high enough to cover the ankle and a non-slip sole such as vibram type maximize protection against sprains on uneven ground. A variety of commercial ankle braces are available but often these will not fit in the boot. These are not necessary unless someone has recently sprained an ankle, but in that situation they may provide added support to permit walking uneven terrain comfortably and securely.

If you find yourself miles from home on a hunting trip and fallen victim to an ankle injury, your trip can be salvaged if your plan of treatment is decisive and rapidly instituted. It is difficult to tell exactly how severely an ankle is sprained when it initially happens and therefore all sprains should be treated quite aggressively. As soon as possible after the injury if ice is available it can be applied directly to the skin in the form of an ice massage over the tender area at 10 to 15 minute intervals three to four times before going to bed that evening. If you are tent camping or do not have access to ice, substitute packed snow, a plastic bag filled with cold spring water or actually emerse the foot and ankle into a cold stream to obtain a similar effect. Total emersion of the foot should not be for longer than 30 seconds at a time in icy high mountain spring water for fear of circulatory problems in the toes.

Later that evening the foot should be elevated, preferrably above the level of the heart to prevent blood and edema fluid from collecting in the ankle. Don't sit around playing uker with your swollen foot hanging down in a dependent position. If you are going to play cards, move the game closer to your bunk, lie down and prop your foot up on two or three pillows. Likewise the foot should be elevated on pillows when sleeping that night. Before bed, a compression wrap should be applied. An elastic bandage such as an A.C.E. is as indispensible an item as adhesive tape in any hunting camp. The A.C.E. bandage should be wrapped snugly but not too tightly. To provide added local compression and thereby minimize swelling, a folded handkerchief or hunting sock

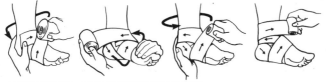

ANKLE WRAP—START ON INSIDE ANKLE

should be placed directly over the injured area beneath the A.C.E. wrap. This selective compressive support will limit the swelling which comes from small bleeding vessels which course through the ankle ligaments that are either stretched or torn. It is the prevention of this swelling that is mandatory so that you can resume early physical activity. Swelling peaks at 24 to 36 hours after an injury. Once swelling is severe, it is very difficult to eliminate. The A.C.E. wrap should remain on all night and the foot should be elevated. If an elastic bandage is not available, one or two pairs of snug fitting support socks can be worn to bed to provide some compression.

I.C.E. (Ice, compression, elevation) program is mainstay that all athletic trainers use for treatment of strains and sprains. Again, its purpose is basically to limit the amount of bleeding and swelling about the injured joint and thereby diminishing the discomfort and allowing earlier motion. The sooner I.C.E. is initiated upon arriving home the more effective it is.

Arising in the morning don't be surprised to find a stiff and sore ankle. There will be some swelling, perhaps even some discoloration over the lateral ankle bone. Sit on the edge of the bed and pump your ankle up and down 10 to 15 times and then take a few steps on it. Walk around the room but before going too far be sure to reapply your A.C.E. wrap snugly if it has been previously removed. Put your boots on before the swelling starts and wear an extra pair of socks or the A.C.E. to maintain compression. Ankle taping should be done only by those who have been trained to do so, such as athletic trainers or therapists.

On your hunt that day stick to unobstructed pathways such as deer trails or logging roads as much as you can. Climbing hills should not be as bothersome as walking on sidehills when your ankle is turned down and in. So if you do have to traverse a sidehill, do so keeping the injured ankle on the uphill side. Walking thus prevents stressing the ligaments that were injured when the foot was turned down and inward. Shorten your stride and slow your pace, remembering that you're a prime risk to resprain the ankle. If there is snow on the ground or damp conditions make the surface slippery it maybe wise to post up for your companion's game drives. Each evening subsequent to your ankle injury it is important to repeat the I.C.E. program until the ankle feels normal again.

One question always arises after an acute ankle sprain; Is my ankle broken? Without an x-ray it is impossible to tell and often times severe sprains appear more swollen, black and blue and even more painful than fractures. If pain persists or worsens, limit your walking, continue the I.C.E. program and see a physician as soon as possible for an x-ray and subsequent treatment. If fractured, the ankle is usually casted for six weeks. The vast majority of ankle injuries however are sprains where the ligaments are stretched excessively or torn. Though not as severe, these injuries can ruin your day or even week or two. If your ankle is prone to injury, preventative measures which include strengthening of the calf muscles and the use of a supportive boot are mandatory. If the ankle is twisted significantly, early aggressive treatment with ice, compression and elevation will limit the swelling, discomfort and provide the best opportunity to early motion and return to protected physical activity afield.

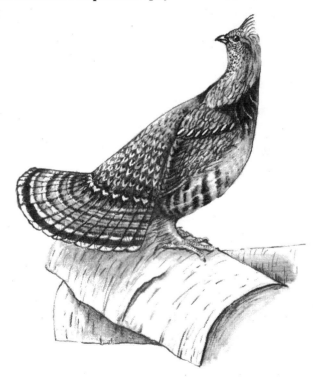

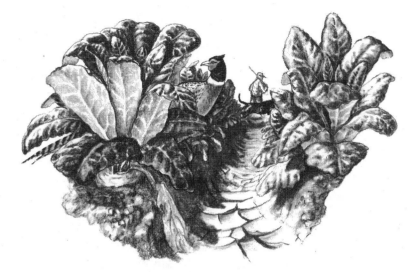

Chapter 10

Knee Sprains
Falling After Beet Field Pheasants

L ast night's unseasonably persistent, pounding rain storm had definitely and effectively cracked summer's record drought, 167 days without a drop. The irrigation ditches like lines of silver tinsel among mounds of deep green beet tops sprawling for acres appeared just partly filled with a slow moving mixture of rain and irrigation water. It lay in waiting.

The seven hour drive north away from the Southern California masses had taken a toll, leaving them both bleary-eyed and exhausted. He and his side-kick, racquetball partner, business associate and all around best man, had decided long ago on the Fourth of July to escape the hustle of L.A. and travel north to the central valley farmland for a week of well deserved and much needed pheasant hunting. Arrangements had been made through a friend of a friend, who happened to own and manage six hundred or so odd acres of prime agricultural land, a proverbial checker board of saffron, sun flowers, corn, beets, and rice all at various stages of harvesting.

The simple frame cottage-like structure that housed itinerant workers during spring and summer provided more than adequate accommodations and as luck would have it, the farmer was able to take a few days from his hectic schedule and join them as guide, hunter, and story teller extraordinaire adding a special touch of local color.

The morning broke early with storm clouds blowing eastward over the coastal range and blue skies trailing in the west. After a night's comalike sleep they awoke early, approached the day optimistically, but had to agree that conditions promised to be far from ideal. In the immediate vicinity grain crops of saffron, sunflower and corn had recently been harvested leaving very little cover in which pheasants could hide. The soggy beet fields were obvious concentration points. There were at least two hundred acre sections in which the pheasants could hide and seek protection.

In the early morning sun the fields appeared massive as long low lines of mud with an occasional pool of water dotted heavily with the green and yellow beet tops protruding from the bowling ball sized sugar beets. It amazed him to briefly contemplate just what would happen with so many sugar beets, realizing that this was only one small plot of this important cash crop in the central valley. Sugar bowls of America were certain to be filled.

Since moving to California a brief six years ago, each fall brought with it thoughts of the northeastern hunting seasons he had known in his earlier life. The differences should have been obvious, but the thought of hunting ringnecks in beet fields with blue skies and eighty-five degree weather, wearing shorts, short-sleeves and a vest with a heavy dose of 15 sun-block smeared on the face still seemed an odd way to approach a day afield. Gone was the need for vibrim soles (they rapidly within four steps collected eighteen pounds of mud), nylon chaps (they fry your legs in the sun), and heavy canvas hunting coat (not needed here for breaking wind or thorns). What mattered now was lightweight, waterproof footwear, cotton trousers, a T-shirt, vest and desire and energy to run after the labradors as they splashed through the damp cover like so many snorting water buffalo in pursuit of the wiley ringneck. The trick is to have a dog blessed with an incomparable nose, then it's up to you to stay close.

The shots will come but the question is range, for pheasants are not so difficult to hit as to hit hard enough to bring down. A California pheasant can absorb even a well placed shot at a distance, and once hit, they're masters at the creep and disappear game making a canine retriever of paramount importance. All of which makes for much sloshing and sucking wind for dog and and hunter alike.

In this region, the world's farming technology capitol, I am sure the plant researchers, botanists, and farmers have calculated to the centimeter just how far apart to plant each beet seed and to mound each row to maximize yield. The fact is that the laser disked rows are too close for a normal and comfortable step from row to row and too far apart to make skipping a row with a giant step feasible. The resultant gait is kind of a short step dance or sliding jog trying to plant your foot firmly between the rotund beets, maintain balance and keep from sliding forward or backward into the muddy foot deep irrigation ditch on either side of the beet row. It goes beyond athletic ability and into the realm of acrobatics, slipping, sliding and balancing between the mounds of beets. To the uneducated eye or non-hunter, our party of five which included a welcome pair of unexpected neighbors and three labradors, no doubt appeared a wavering line of grown men recently deep in touch with John Barleycorn, floundering after a few wild and crazy dogs, bent on tearing apart some huge spinach patch.

The fact that everyone knows they should take short choppy steps, and with extreme caution does not prevent the inevitable. Buck, one monstrous black lab was trying to figure out some double helix configuration escape path of a running rooster. Suddenly he stopped short, spun 190 degrees and made a quick lunge to the right, flushing a cock bird from between his paws. Back pedaling, side-stepping and trying to close the gap between frantic man and frantic dog his left foot failed to negotiate one extra large sugar beet. Rather than plant firmly, his foot struck on an angle, then violently slipped down and back uncontrollably into the muddy ditch. With his body's momentum moving forward and slipping foot moving backward something gave within the knee with resounding snap as it hyperextended and rotated. Within a fraction of a second he hit the ground in a heap.

Falling to the wet clay soil, he knew immediately something major had shifted inside his knee. Surprising himself, he arose without much discomfort and brushed the mud from his jeans. Walking took extreme concentration and effort and there was some pain, but not as much as he would have imagined as he managed to slowly maneuver himself back to the car. By that time his entire leg felt like a thick rubber band. He had little control of his leg and it felt like it might buckle at every step. He sat on the front seat with the car door open trying to "work out" whatever had happened.

The haunting chant of his high school football coach, the guy who disapproved of pain, came welling up to him, "walk it off, work it out." Try as he might he could do neither. By the time the rest of his party had collected the last two birds to ultimately fill their limit then straggled back to the car, his knee felt stiff and swollen. Pain was present now deep within the knee, but was not severe. Still he did not trust his leg would support him when he tried to walk on it. To protect it from buckling he locked his knee as straight as he could in a stifflegged limp and by that evening when they set out to dinner there were comments all around about Matt Dillion's old side kick Chester from Dodge City. He failed to be amused. Before bedtime, the swelling was severe as the knee filled with fluid (blood as he was to find out later) and was uncomfortable to flex or extend. He knew at that point that unless some miracle passed his way through this intermittent and itinerant abode tonight while sleeping, his central valley pheasant hunt was over.

A restless night's sleep did nothing to improve the stiffness, swelling, and discomfort, and if anything had changed, it was yet a more apprehensive feeling that his knee just simply would not hold him. Mad as a hatter, he packed up and headed home. Eventually he was emotionally, then physically forced into his doctor's office by his long suffering family after a week of "it will get better by itself."

He had torn one of the main ligaments of the knee, the anterior cruciate ligament. He underwent a surgical arthroscopy so that the orthopedist could visualize the damage inside the knee particularly the cruciate ligament and remove a small portion of torn cartilage (meniscus) that happened simultaneously with the ligament tear. His recovery and rehabilitation was lengthy in terms of weeks, but successful and he was back chasing pheasants the next season, but now staying out of wet fields and on damp days wearing a special brace that supported his knee just as his cruciate ligament once did.

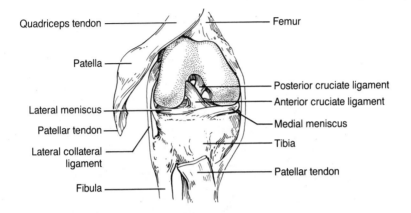

All this from a slip and twist? All this and more. In competitive athletics twisting and hyperextension injuries to the knee often times result in severe damage to the joint rendering it excessively loose, many times requiring ligament repair, reconstruction or cartilage removal. This unfortunate injury occurs all too frequently and despite all of the sports medicine research efforts to prevent the injury, the incidence remains high. The severity of injury can usually be determined early by the rapid onset of swelling in the knee which in actuality is bleeding, however, it is at times difficult to tell whether it is a ligament or cartilage tear or both. If this unfortunate accident occurs, it is important to have it evaluated by your physician soon so that a correct diagnosis and treatment plan can be instituted early.

Once the type of damage is documented, the knee rarely returns to normal. That is not to say that you cannot become functional and pain free after an extensive exercise program to strengthen the thigh muscles, but the knee may always feel slightly loose. If the muscles are strong they can dynamically stabilize the joint but if they are not, the knee is at extreme risk for a reinjury. The hamstrings, the muscles in the back of the thigh, are most important and can be strengthened by knee curls with a weight machine or free weights lying face down with the weight hooked behind the heel and the knee then is bent upward ninety degrees. Power is an important aspect of rehabilitation from this injury and therefore heavy weights (thirty to fifty pounds) should eventually be used in sets of ten repetitions. The quadriceps, likewise, are vital to knee stability and can be strengthened by sitting with the weight suspended from the front of the ankle and thus the knee is extended again in sets of ten repetitions (refer to Figure 2-7). A similar poundage should be used for knee curls and extensions. Leg presses and wall squats use both quads and hams simultaneously and are also beneficial.

If the knee is extremely loose and continues to give out, then a special brace may be prescribed to provide stability. In extreme cases, this ligament which notoriously is a poor healer, needs to be reconstructed with extensive surgery.

Cartilage is much easier to deal with for its presence is not nearly as vital to knee function. If a cartilage tear is present, it is removed or repaired by arthroscopic means. Rehabilitation is rapid, and the hunter stands a good chance of chasing game within four weeks after a removal. Arthroscopic techniques now permit repair of certain meniscal tears. But longer protection in terms of months is required following a repair.

Many men who suffered knee injuries playing ball in high school or college still may be troubled by a "trick knee," thereby exhibiting long standing ligament or cartilage damage. Remarkably they have compensated and adapted to this usually significant disability by modifing their activities. They are usually unimpeded in their routine daily lives, but when their activity level increases to say hill climbing or walking slippery turf, pain or noticeable swelling may occur within the knee and at this point it is time to have it evaluated. The swelling or "water-on-the-knee" is a more significant indicator of irritation and on going injury, than is pain. It is certain that this knee will not get better by itself but can often times be made better by simple surgery or even by an aggressive rehabilitation exercise program.

No one likes to visit the doctor, but then again, no one wants to give up hunting either, we all want durability from our bodies and quality time afield. Modern orthopedic technology now permits evaluation of acute or chronic knee injuries by scans or special x-ray tests, and arthroscopy whereby a magnifying telescope the size of a pencil, can be inserted into the knee under regional anesthsia. The knee then, can be thoroughly visualized and the majority of times, the problem can be corrected by using small, fine instruments through minute incisions done as an out-patient procedure.

The point is that if you have had an old knee injury and continue to have a trick knee that is slowing you down or has stopped your excursions all together, have it evaluated and at least get on a rehabilitation exercise program. It often times can be the difference between hunting with gusto or hunting at all.

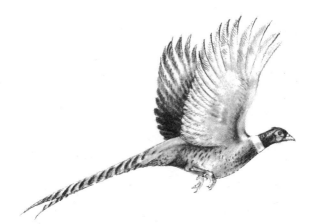

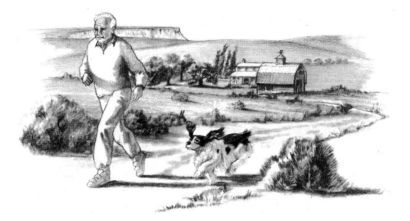

Chapter 11

The Aging Hunter

The alarm sounded from somewhere across the blackened room like an irritating squal from the depth of a cave. He lay there briefly remembering what is soon to come—opening day ducks on the Mississippi bottoms. Rapid, mind sharp glimpses of greenhead wedges suspended above the blocks pervade his drowsiness. It's time now to rise and take them. The bounce out of bed now is no longer graceful and there is a swagger to the sink for a quick splash of cold water in the face. The joints take a few laps around the kitchen to loosen up. Soon the mind and body are both ready and facing the day with excitement and confidence.

After a morning rush of teal and an occasional wood duck the sun stood high signalling the predicted cessation of flight. Today he felt like one true hunting gentleman, mystifying his young nephew with luring teal whistles and then dropping a few bluewings at 50 yards after his young cohort shot holes all around the fleeing birds. Yes, he still had it, and he felt strong and self assured. The sun's warmth was comforting as he entered the phase of duck hunting, older and more experienced hunters call casual reconnaissance which could be done with the eyes open or closed if you had a good dog to let you know that some mallards silently dropped in and were now swimming fearlessly about the decoys. Casual reconnaissance, most veteran duck hunters swore, preserved energy for the evening flight and it provided savory time to let the mind wander back in time.

He had hunted the flyway now for well over fifty years but each opening day brought back the thrill of seasons past like flipping a switch on his mind's black and white movie newsreel. There was his first greenhead drake, taken quite by chance as it hovered over his grandfather's hand carved blocks. He pointed the old Parker skyward, closed his eyes and prayed as he pulled the trigger. The naive feeling of arrogance lasted only briefly that morning and then came the painful humility of being lucky. Humility was figuratively and effectively pounded into his head after shooting four or five more boxes of shells through the big double until finally he scored again much later that season. Perhaps he had arrived.

He once again felt the icy water from many years ago envelop him in a shocking chill as he rapidly tore off his hip boots and hunting jacket and dove headlong into the Mississippi's high brown current in an attempt to rescue his young golden retriever that couldn't say no to a wingshot bluebill. Disregarding his owner's commands the pup broke free at the sight of the downed duck only to eventually become tangled in a morass of lily pads. As the young dog struggled the tentacles of the water vines dragged him beneath the powerful river current beside the main channel and ended his brief but valiant life. He remembered the grief of losing his young companion but was thankful that day for his own strength and decisiveness that allowed him to realize his life was also in jeopardy and return to the island, frigid, exhausted, and resigned that he could not help save his dog. Tears welled up in the cups of his eyes as he thought about other dogs that had shared his blinds, each one a singular personality. Each one taught him more in general about being free in the outdoors and specifically about the art of duck hunting. Soft nostalgia was an acceptable and even desireable benefit of aging.

He had seen the cycles in duck population with wing filled skies of the late forties and early fifties which allowed large bag limits, to the downswing drought years of the seventies when once popular ducks such as the black and woodies were rarely seen and bag limits became quite sparse. It didn't seem to matter any more, the bag limit that is. When he was younger it seemed important to always fill out your limit. Retrospectively he considered himself at that time somewhat of a meat hunter, but acknowledges this a sign of youth in the vein of "more is better." Now, though it was nice to return home with a brace of healthy sprig, or occasional honker and it was the quality of the event along with the pomp, preparation, and companionship that created and maintained his enjoyment.

Most of his snoring companions were of the next generation and hopefully not the last that would experience similar outdoor adventures. He remembered youthful times when he and his companions stayed up at night in Mike's old boat house down by Buck's slough, or often in their jon boat beached beside their blind, playing cards by the hissing light of the Coleman lantern. He could not remember now exactly why it was necessary to stay up all night but more likely than not it was one of those manly things to do at the time. His body now rebelled with less than eight hours sleep each night and as so often happens when one grows up, the mind becomes accustomed to the body, and he listens to what his body tells him and responds accordingly.

The process of aging is a phenomenon that no one understands entirely, but everyone would like it to slow down or stop. And yet like the rising of the sun it progresses at its own rate with no regard to individual whims. Aging theoretically begins at the end of adolescence, around age twenty. It is a gradual maturing of the body, a slowing down of biological processes and thus, an overall reduction of human cellular and chemical performance. That is not to say that life is a downhill slide and crash after age 25. We all know and have hunted with senior partners twice our age and not only marvel at their skill and endurance but often times find ourselves shamefully unable to keep their pace. Suffice to say, individuals age at different rates and it remains difficult to correlate physiological or functional age with chronological age which is the actual time spent on this planet. We do know in generic terms that many physiological changes do occur in a relative pattern as everyone lives and learns to get a grip on life.

For many, aging means losing; losing the obvious such as hair, hearing, sight and perhaps libido. The rate of decline or loss varies from tissue to tissue and individual to individual. Changes occur slowly, the most noticeable perhaps, lies in the realm of the musculoskeletal system. This kinetic chain of bones, joints and muscles not only supports internal organs but also propels us along in search of game. Scientific studies have shown that after age 25 the average man will subsequently lose approximately 1% of his muscle strength per year or to state more simply, at age 50 you will have lost 25% and therefore will theoretically be only three/fourths as strong as your peak strength at age 25. This estimated decline in strength appears more noticable in the trunk and legs than in the arms, because in our American society, most people use their upper extremities at work or around the home whereas very few daily activities demand much from our abdominal, back, or leg muscles.

A classic example would be a dairy farmer, who is up at five a.m. milking his Holsteins as he has for the past thirty-five years, throwing hay bales and then mounting his green John Deere and riding off into the sunrise for a day of plowing, cutting, or harvesting. Many of my farmer friends, even in their sixties, continue this rigorous daily activity and not one would I engage in an arm wrestling contest for their hands, forearms, and upper arms have evolved into massive power instruments. On the other hand, many of these same individuals that can lift a small barn have trouble walking very far or climbing hills. Strong, absolutely, but very selectivly so and only in the arms, but their leg and trunk strength as well as aerobic endurance remains average at best.

Other physiological aspects of muscle aging are actually more important to the hunter than maximum strength and these involve neuromuscular coordination, reaction time, and endurance. For muscles to work, individual nerves must fire electrical impulses within each muscle fiber causing the contraction and coordination of these contractions resulting in a precise movement of the limb. The aging process slows down the transmission of this impulse from the brain down through the nerve. Likewise when the muscle contracts, a retrograde impulse from the muscle back to the brain lets it know that movement is complete and the muscle is ready for another stimulation. This series of inputs and feedbacks occurs in milliseconds, without conscious thought, and allows for complex and coordinated movement.

The older hunter might recognize this phenomenon when traversing uneven ground. Not as quick and steady on your feet as you once were and you do not feel as confident bouncing along at the rapid clip as you once did. Without recognizing this fact and bailing out in a head long charge over untested ground, this hunter is a set up for injury. In such a situation protection must come by slowing down the pace or taking shorter strides and on occasions, making a conscious effort to "read" the footing beneath you. It is also possible to maintain one's neuromuscular coordination by practice and training. In your off season fitness program, add exercises that demand a bit more agility such as rope jumping (not just for sissies), jumping jacks (emphasizing different positions of foot placement), hopping (either single leg or box hopping from a low stable platform such as the floor to a higher one such as a porch, deck or stair [Figure 11-1]) and even running backwards and sideways.

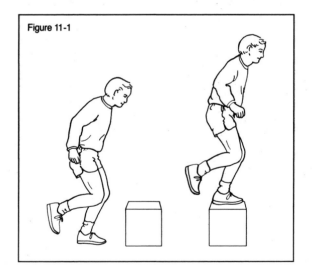

Figure 11-1

Along with coordination runs reaction time, the speed with which a group of muscles or the entire body reacts to a given stimulus such as the thunderous explosion of a pair of grouse. Reaction time initially involves one or more of the five senses, usually sight or sound followed by foot placement for support, positioning of the trunk, rapid but flowing motion of the arms bringing the shotgun up to the sighting eye, finally tracking and swinging until the bird is overtaken, the proper lead established and shot is taken. Aging slows this reaction time. Most game birds fly thirty to fifty miles an hour and provide but three to five seconds for this entire process to occur and each decade the shooter must make some adjustments to compensate for his slowing reaction time. Simply lifting weights will help. How much does your shotgun weigh, six or seven pounds? So you do not have to be a power lifter to shoulder and swing a shotgun, but it certainly helps maintain reaction time to use five or ten pound dumbbells for some rapid repetition curls, presses, and flies. Jogging or walking with hand or wrist weights occasionally is even more functional and specific to shooting. Racquet sports like tennis or squash or jabbing at a punching bag will aid reaction time. The nerves and muscles of the body respond not only to the amount of work they do by hypertrophying but also to the speed at which they work. Therefore bouts of rapid but light weight lifting is an important adjunct to add to preseason conditioning. Intensity training or imaging will also boost your senses by making them more aware of the first wing beat thereby starting this reaction process earlier.

In the confines of your den or study and when the family is at the movies, practice your mount, swing and point with your favorite shotgun. Snap shooting the corners of your room a few minutes a week gives a smoother feel for the shotgun swing and its sighting plane. Nothing puts it all together in pre-season, however, like actually shooting clay birds, not however, in typical fashion with a gun at shoulder mount from the cement circle of a trap range. Leave the trap house after a few rounds to sharpen the eyes and get into the woods where the real birds will be. A trusted friend with a hand trap and a backpack full of clay pigeons walking through a wooded area much better simulates hunting conditions. The thrower, from behind or to the side, stops at undesignated times, yells, and launches the yellow and black clay directly toward the old white pine or through an opening in the aspen grove and you must react before the branches and boughs gobble up the bird. New founded enthusiasm for sporting clays has been encouraging for this type of shooting is based again on hunting situations.

Like coordination, agility, and reaction time our muscular endurance likewise fades as the years mount. Muscular endurance, repetitive muscle contraction without fatigue, is what keeps us going all day. Endurance remains more vital to us for overall performance than does maximum strength and can be thought of simply as the art of pacing oneself. Once this art is recognized and practiced endurance can be maintained at a rather steady state with minimal decline compared to strength or agility which gradually digress despite our efforts. Like the other neuromuscular elements, endurance is best maintained by practice, performing repeated submaximal efforts in the form of some type of resistance weight training or aerobic exercise like walking. The ideal length of time to practice this act of fitness has not been determined, but relates directly to the demands that you place upon your body. If you are planning on half-day hunts throughout the season, brisk daily walks of one half to one hour a day and light weight lifting three times a week should be adquate to maintain endurance and prevent fatigue for your half day hunts. On the other hand, if you are planning a full season hunting daily for six to eight hours, then a more demanding endurance conditioning schedule is necessary.

Some older hunters, whether they are retired or on vacation, push themselves into strenuous daily hunts. Usually after three or four days of this, the body becomes reluctant and at times rebellious and what ordinarily would seem enjoyable feels much more like work. When conditioning endurance athletes such as marathoners or triathletes, we encourage alternating hard and soft days, the hard days being longer in terms of time and mileage and the demands higher in terms of speed or muscular effort, the short being just the opposite. It is also recommended that at least one and possibly two days of relative rest are taken during the week to allow the body to rejuvenate itself. The point is when planning a season or even a one week hunt, scatter a few casual, more restful days among those with heavy demand and your trip will be much more enjoyable.

For the normal person with routine exercise, the cardiovascular system reaches a stable, steady state and for the older, healthy hunter is rarely the limiting factor when out in the field. More often it is fatigue of other body muscles and joint discomfort that slow you down rather than the huffing, puffing and difficulty catching your breath. Aging of the cardiovascular system is inevitable and well established are the factors that accelerate this process, often times to a pathological and dangerous degree.

These cardiac risk factors are heredity or family history of heart attacks, smoking, high blood pressure, obesity, high blood cholesterol, and sedentary lifestyle. The presence of even one factor increases the possibility of a heart attack. It becomes clear then that the overweight, 45 year old, smoking, business executive whose father dies of a myocardial infarction at age 50 may be risking his life each exerted effort when hunting. Of all the cardiac risk factors, the only one we have no control over is our hereditary constitution. The remainder are manageable and deserve our attention and manipulation at times. Maintaining a healthy heart means limiting or eliminating those controllable risk factors and a simple scientifically proven way to do that is participating in some form of aerobic exercise. Studies have shown that aerobic conditioning for twenty to thirty minutes at least three times a week will: lower blood cholesterol, aid in weight loss, lower hypertension, and even diminish the desire to smoke. The well conditioned heart muscle contracts more efficiently and has better circulation within itself. The key to initiating a safe fitness program in middle age is to pursue a gradual progression of exercise and more importantly consistency in participation.

Body metabolism slows down as we grow older. Metabolism can be thought of as the efficiency with which all of the body's cells operate. We no longer need the high octane fuel to maintain our energy levels. Those of us who have raised adolescents know that teenagers seem to be constantly starving while eating their way from here to Texas and usually not gaining any weight at all in the process. Where are they putting it all? The cells in their bodies are using this high calorie intake not only for growth but also are operating at a much faster rate.

After age 25, it is important to rethink the weight maintenance equation (body weight = calories consumed - calories expended). For such a slow down in body processes will diminish the caloric burn-up and if we do not respond by lowering our intake or increasing our activity output, weight gain, even to a point of obesity, becomes a very real possibility. Excessive weight not only puts extra strain on heart function but also creates tremendous reaction forces across the joints resulting in accelerated cartilage wear thereby increasing the possibility of arthritis. If an overweight individual is having musculoskeletal pains with activity, merely bringing their weight down to within 10% of ideal body weight lessens the strain and resultant wear. To put this in biomechanical terms, a 10 pound weight loss results in a 40 pound reduction of joint reaction force across the knee during heavy walking activities.

If you already have some degree of joint arthritis, your hunt can be made less agonizing simply by taking a couple of aspirin or your favorite anti-inflammatory pill an hour before going out. This will not just deaden pain that you might experience, rather it diminishes the arthritic inflammation of the joints, lessens the congestion thereby limiting swelling and pain during and particularly after the hunt. Most anti-inflammatory pills initiate action in one hour and are effective for approximately four hours so you may wish to take a couple aspirin along with you for lunch. Remember that aspirin can cause gastritis (stomach burning) in some people. This side effect can be lessened by using a buffered compound or taking the pills with food or antacids.

For the arthritic hunter, plan your hunt to be less physically demanding early and late in the day thereby providing warm-up and cool down situations. In the off season it is mandatory to maintain musculoskeletal coordination, reaction time, and endurance, to improve performance but more importantly, strong muscles act as shock absorbers for the joints. Shock absorbers in lousy condition fail to protect our joints from high impact forces and the wearing process accelerates.

Aging is not all gloom and doom and there are many benefits to growing up. One that comes with years and experience, often overlooked, is simple common sense. Pacing yourself particularly the first hour in the morning to allow warm-up time makes sense. Likewise, periodic rests of ten minutes and perhaps even a brief nap in mid-afternoon beneath your favorite pine tree, allows time for recovery. Hunting can either be a social event or an introspective adventure in solitude. Hunting alone, one controls his own pace. Pacing can also be attained by hunting with a partner your own age or with similar physical attributes. When out with young, hard chargers, they hopefully will be sensitive to your slow but steady pace, but if not, a quick review of your favorite gun dog training book will come in handy as you educate your young "man-dog" to the fine arts of breaking brush or making game in the prickly ash. It is important for them to scout likely looking ridge tops while you guard the logging trails. It's mandatory they hold still while you work your way into shooting position at the edge of a cattail swamp. Expending his energy and saving yours while passing on your wealth of knowledge and art of harvesting game — quite a deal and it is the crafty man who can pull it off and still maintain a heroe's stance.

These guidelines followed, there is no reason to think of yourself as over the hill and fading fast and certainly not hanging up your gun and forgetting hunting altogether. Remember, although physical prowess declines with age, wisdom and sage ascend. It is a wise hunter who realizes his limitations and his attributes and practices to maintain them.

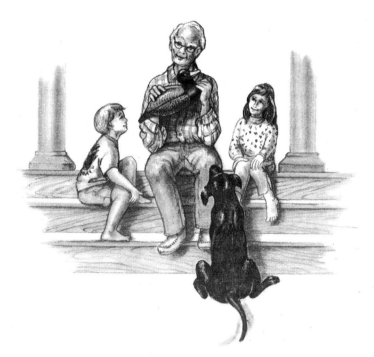

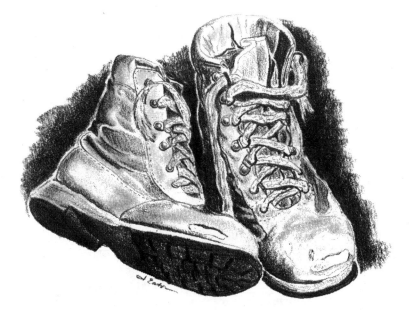

Chapter 12

The Hunter's Achille's Heel
Pain in the Foot

It hurts to say good-bye to an old friend, reliving all the good times and conveniently forgetting the bad. That is the feeling, like burying your favorite setter. The ragged, torn, and ancient boots are gently lowered into the trashcan. The lid closes on the passing of an era. Those boots cost eighteen ninety-five a few years back, well maybe sixteen or so, and during that time they've been in the service of protecting and providing for poor feet in all conditions, terrain, and weather. They have been restitched at least three times and resoled a half a dozen. They kept going when I thought I couldn't, but the years have finally taken their toll. The once sturdy and amazingly comfortable pair over the years had been molded and macerated into structureless clumps of leather and rubber a consistency of a doe-skinned slipper with a foam sole. No longer was there cushion against the ground, nor was there stout support for the ankles not to mention their more recent sieve-like waterproof qualities that developed within the last few years. Their condition had become so deplorable that the last year or so each day afield meant a night in a water tub, soaking, sometimes hot and sometimes cold, but always directed at the bruised and blistered beings at the ends of my legs. At times if it weren't for the snow, I might have found barefeet a more functional and less painful approach. But I loved them.

Everyone can think back to the day when you had finally saved enough money to purchase your first pair of classic boots, be they bird shooters, Irish setters, or leather pacs. With certainty this eventful purchase could be justified by doing what the masters did and then by magical transference your aim would be sharper and no doubt more game would find its way to the table. Often times it seems the uniform of hunting is that which makes one a better shot. Hero worship, boot buying aside, these legendary foot covers did provide the basis for future functional footwear.

Breaking nostalgia is always a difficult, and at times dangerous thing to do to sportsmen, but if the truth can be told, many of the age old boot classics were actually hard on the feet. Though beautifully hand stitched and feeling like a cloud when they were worn in the shoe store, the story changed dramatically with terrain not nearly as soft and smooth as carpet especially after a season or two of hard wear. Nostalgia slows the winds of change, but change is now blowing through the sporting boot world. The brand names may be the prestigous same or a relative newcomer, but the boot is very different and this is much to the hunter's advantage.

The changes in shoeware in the past five to ten years can be directly correlated with the national fervor for fitness and jogging in particular. There was a time not so long ago that the Converse canvas high tops were the top line athletic shoes, but today that shoe is appreciated much like a dinosaur for the cushioning material was rigid gum-rubber, the forefoot sole flexibility was inconsistent and canvas uppers provided no support whatsoever for the ankle.

In the late 1960's, physicians, biomechanists, and runners

themselves began analyzing the runner's foot. For people to run five to ten miles everyday was a new phenomenon for the recreational athlete, but for the hunter this mileage was old hat. The function of the foot is much better understood now and not to understate it, the foot is a remarkable linkage of bones and tendons that must be a flexible shock absorber when the foot first hits the ground at heel strike. Then it must transform itself into a rigid lever arm that provides a base for the muscles and tendons to pull against thereby propelling the entire body forward by toe-off. It has further been shown that because of the ground reaction force, the foot at each step is subjected to forces at least two to three times that of body weight with walking and as high as six times body weight when running. By controlling these tremendous forces at the foot level it prevents the shock and wear from being transferred further up the leg to other vital weight bearing joints like the knee and hip.

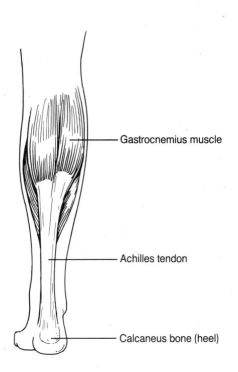

Gastrocnemius muscle

Achilles tendon

Calcaneus bone (heel)

The evolution of the running shoe has been an interesting course to follow. In the early seventies, each year brought one more item of refinement, one more bit of biomechanical information that was translated into the shoe not only to improve performance, but also to prevent injuries. Many fine points still stir controversy, but such is the competitive business of shoe marketing. There are basic elements of footwear that remain constant and by applying many of the running shoe concepts, today's hunting boots are running closely on the coattails of the athletic shoe technology.

The basics for functional sport boots include: 1) a well cushioned heel to absorb ground reaction force at heel strike, 2) rear foot support with rigid heel counters to prevent excessive side to side motion of the foot and in some cases, more sturdy uppers to help stabilize the ankle, 3) a flexible sole to prevent excessive strain and overuse of the Achilles' tendon, foot, and calf muscles that push off, and 4) appropriate length and width of the toe box to prevent blisters, cramps, and in some individuals painful bunions.

Once again it is important not to be lured into the shoe store comfort of a boot. Early in the evolution of running shoes we learned that simply building up layers of soft cushion soles that initially felt so comfortable actually became the foot's worst enemy. With wear the sole became unstable thereby providing a shifting base when the foot was planted. If a person has ideal biomechanical structure of the foot these ultra soft shoes are acceptable but for most of us, however, with relatively abnormal foot structure this soft shifting base soon creates abnormal wear patterns, break down of the heel counter and forefoot of the shoe and eventually leads to foot pain. Therefore the ideal sports boot has a balance between softness in the heel and sole and structural rigidity to control the foot. This is particularly true if the hunter has flat feet or foot pronation.

For those hunters with severe pronation some companies are now applying advanced athletic technology, fashioning their boots with a variably compressive heel, molded with a thin flexible sole. To this they have applied a thin, lightweight vibram outer sole (from mountain climbing technology) for grip and slip protection. The heel counters are rigid and toe box ample . Certain companies even provide orthotic type inserts (arch supports) for added support for the pronating foot. The end result is a boot that controls the foot not only at heel strike but throughout the entire gait cycle until the toe leaves the ground.

Foot afflictions in hunters are numerous. There are yet a few Southern gentlemen and a number of big game hunters that still chase their game on horesback and hopefully none of us have fallen into the noisy lure of all-terrain vehicles or motorcycles to transport us to our game. The fact remains that, like it or not, our feet have been and always will be our main source of transportation while hunting. Foot afflictions vary widely from blisters and heel pain to arch strain and tendonitis and if one of these problems becomes severe it matters not if you are in great physical shape, you only make it as far as your closest deer stand.

At the risk of approaching first-aid suggestion and hopefully common sense, a few thoughts about blisters are warranted. This, the most common foot injury, results from friction. Excessive rubbing and sliding of two surfaces against one another creates heat. Blister formation however is more complex than simply a thermal burn. Blisters actually form due to the shearing forces between the outer skin (epidermis) and the inner layer or dermis. A small tear between the two becomes a cleft filled with inflammatory extracellular fluid. These are the nasty red fluid filled blebs that cause such grief on the heels and toes.

Friction can be limited obviously by wearing proper boot size and wearing them enough to break in both the boot and the foot. This time of mutual adaptation between boot and foot should begin briefly, perhaps only an hour and then gradually the time worn is extended. As the foot is subjected to friction and pressure at different prominent points, the skin will thicken, forming protective calluses and therefore be less likely to blister.

Friction can also be transferred away from the foot and to the socks if worn in layers. Preferrably the inner sock (liner) should be elastically form-fitting, thin and wicking as well as slippery to transfer the friction interface away from the skin and to the socks themselves. Combinations of Spandex, Lycra, or light-weight polypropylene liners worn beneath heavy wool, thermax or thicker polypropylene socks is ideal. These types of lining socks can be purchased in athletic shoe and sport shops.

Blister formation is enhanced by excessive moisture and heat.

Keep your feet dry by limiting perspiration. Spraying feet with deodorant compounds is definitely effective. Liberal doses of talcum powder should also be rubbed over the foot and between the toes the morning before a long walk.

If the blister has already formed, it is best to cleanse it with soap and water or alcohol and remove the entire blister with small scissors to prevent the re-accumulation of fluid. Air should be allowed to dry it out. Before the next hunt, dress it with antiseptic ointment or a hydrogel dressing such as Spenco Second Skin. An adhesive layer of moleskin patch should be applied to cover it completely. Sheets of moleskin can be purchased in most pharmacies, but don't be surprised if you have to search a bit to find it. I'll never forget my Alaskan, Resurrection Trail blisters, stacked three high, as I hobbled into the one and only general store at trail's end and asked painfully for some moleskin. The lady proprietor dropped her jaw and retorted, "You want what kind of skin, honey? We don't skin any moles up here." The point is, take some with you on your outings.

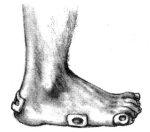

Heel bruise is likely to become troublesome when the ground surface is hard and rocky or if the hunt involves jumping such as over logs or dry creek gullies. Protection and prevention of this sharp, nagging pain involves extra heel cushions such as Spenco or Sorbothane. If the heel pain is associated with an arch strain, a plastic heel cup is helpful.

The combination of heel and arch pain is called plantar fasciitis. It is a form of tendinitis and typically is first noticed and most aggravating when the hunter arises from bed in the morning. Stepping out of bed his heel feels like he is stepping on a stone until he gently walks around the room a few times and the foot warms up. The pattern then is for the pain to gradually resolve at least to a tolerable degree as long as the person is moving and active, but after resting an hour or so, the pain returns immediately when weight is borne on the foot. Plantar fasciitis is usually associated with people who have a very high-arched foot or one that is extremely flat. Tightness of the calf and foot muscles also puts one at risk to develop this inflammatory strain. Prevention and treatment is provided by stretching the calf and foot muscles with wall-leans (Figure 12-1) three times a day and by wearing an arch support (orthotic) either off the shelf, such as a Spenco or Dr. Scholl's type or one that is custom made for you by your physician. Strengthening the calf and foot muscles with toe raises and rope jumping later helps prevent or rehabilitate this condition.

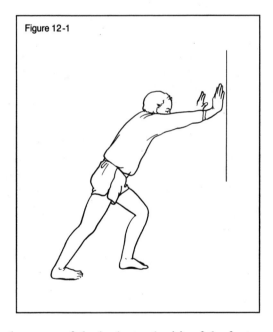

Figure 12-1

As in other parts of the body, tendonitis of the foot occurs when the muscles and tendons are overused in an attempt to dynamically stabilize a foot which is too rigid or too flat. It can also be simply a result of overuse or pushing off too many times in one day. The Achilles tendon or heel cord is most often involved. This cord attaches the calf muscles to the back of the heel and provides the push that propels you from foot flat to toe-off. When the Achilles is inflammed or strained there is usually swelling and tenderness to touch and attempting to stand on your tiptoes hurts severely. If, however, you have experienced one episode of significant injury such as a fall or a forceful toe off with the foot, the Achilles tendon itself can tear. It usually does so with a pop and a feeling that someone has kicked you or thrown a stone at your heel cord or calf. That night the swelling will be significant and it will soon turn black and blue. You will be able to walk, but you will not be able to push off nor stand on your toes comfortably. The unfortunate individual is usually 35-55 years of age. Unlike calf muscle strains, tears of the actual tendon demand physician attention and usually surgical repair for adequate healing in active people.

For simple tendinitis, the rest-ice-compression-elevation (R.I.C.E.) program is initiated early on and followed by wall-lean stretching and muscle conditioning toe raises and jump ropes as symptoms subside. A one quarter inch heel lift fashioned from felt, dense foam, or leather can be used to alleviate pain while walking. Spend the next day or two walking flat terrain if possible as a strong and pain-free Achilles is mandatory for climbing hills. Start aspirin early for best effect.

The foot is often overlooked as a source of disability, but when one analyzes the punishment that it takes day in and day out, mile after mile, it is really not surprising. Prevention of foot problems starts with selecting a boot that combines balance, support, and cushioning. Conditioning exercises are necessary to maintain flexibility and strengthen the calf and foot muscles to prevent overuse tendinitis and strains. And finally, for those who have problems with their arches or other biomechanical and structural defects various over-the-counter pads, cups, lifts, and arch supports are available and effective.

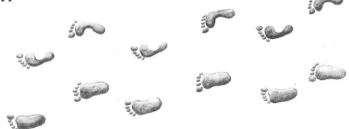

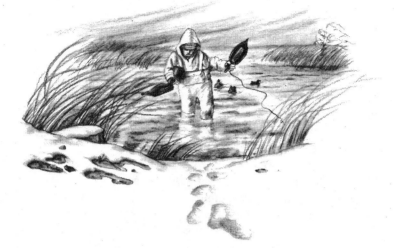

Chapter 13

Chilled to the Bone

Brisk was not the word. Brisk stops at the skin and just inside the nasal passage. This was more a chill, to the depths of the lungs and to the marrow of the bone. And to think it all started out so balmy, as last night's November stars twinkled relentlessly until grey light of dawn gave way to a red rim around the east bay. Forty-five degrees, but the forecaster promised a rapidly approaching noreaster to dampen the day for most inhabitants of New England and eastern Canada, except for those few wise old duck hunters whose skiffs and flats have been impatiently waiting all fall for this event. The big northern push, as it comes suddenly out of the Artic, like a huge icy hand, prodding the reluctant rafts of the scaup and whistlers ahead as the wind whips the bays into frozen froth and soon, in certain areas, solid ice.

Wrapped in long johns, woolen shirt and sweater and draped with his extra large and extra ancient canvas coat he felt overdressed and too warm in the early darkness. But, as the 18 foot punt headed into the wind towards the rocky island destination, he buckled his gloves, buttoned his neck up and pulled down his flannel ear muffs, tying them tightly beneath his chin. He told himself that he would be warm again very shortly after the twenty minute cruise. The salty taste of the sea found his tongue with a reverse drool as the salt spray damped his moustache and everything else from head to toe. It was with a sigh of relief that he crawled over the bow when it struck the rocky shore and clamored, hip boots and all, over the slippery shore line, pulling the line to secure their boat.

There was something omninous about the calm in the air, but for now, he felt comfortable. They temporarily tied their camouflaged punt to a basketball size granite boulder and picked their way to the tip of a long arm of the island that jutted out westward into the bay, like a rock strewn spit. By the red rim of dawn they gathered stones, sparce beams and branches of driftwood from the shoreline and struck their home blind for the day. For these two waterfowlers, this still remained the most exciting and entertaining part of the duck hunting. Some enjoyed arranging and rearranging decoys, like searching for a missing piece in some waterfowl jigsaw puzzle. Others, looked forward to cozy camaraderie in a permanent blind, complete with space heater, propane stove, and poker game. Still others just couldn't wait for the morning flight and the chance to shower the sky with steel balls, the more the better, in hope that some unlucky duck might fly into a charge. It's the action that counts.

Blind building is an acceptable extension of childhood and of the hundreds of shacks that he and his friends used to build as children. It all went by the books, first choosing the proper location, using only local items in construction, then keeping the profile low and uncluttered so as not to attract attention. The principal was concealment. Keep it simple and if it was comfortable, that was merely a bonus. Today's blind sat on the tip of the spit, facing west. A shallow gravelike form took shape as the polished sea stones were piled around to add a slight elevation to the walls. Concealment, not comfort, was priority. A few small driftwood branches washed ashore were braced with rocks and used as a rough shod bench.

The launch was untied and walked through the shallows to the tip of the spit. The wind arose suddenly as the bluebill blocks were dropped in a long line, starting from the windward side of the point, hooking around to the calmer lee pocket directly in front of the blind. Day had definitely declared itself as the two hunters unwrapped and pitched decoys frantically. The eight dozen or so were mostly handcrafted corks with a few dozen cedar golden eyes that were set up in a group, inconspicuously segregated just to the south of the scaup. In their hurry, both had felt a swell or two just clear the tops of their waders and even with their shirt sleeves rolled high, these likewise eventually became wet with the sea. What the sea did not dampen, their perspiration from the exertion of setting blocks did.

As they dove back into their boulder blind, cold was the farthest thing from their minds. As their hearts raced, large rafts of divers rose, almost as if by some prearranged signal. They wiped the salt spray from their guns and slammed home the three inch magnums, excited, as only two duck hunters at daybreak can be. It takes little to appease a duck hunter and it wasn't long before both appreciated sitting and squatting low in their blind, away from the now insistant breeze. Their Chesapeake Bay retriever, a veteran of many such chilly mornings, had spent very little time in the water yet, looked nearly dry and cozy as she sat mesmerized by the trading flights. Where do they come from and where do they all go?

A wedge of broadbills zipped past the point, much too quicky to afford a shot, but at least the pace was set. The mind now quickens; the body warms, as the heart races and the eye and gun instinctively match speeds, anticipating the next flock. It took a moment only, and a half a dozen black and white dive bombers assaulted the cork blocks just outside the quiet ring. The guns sounded and a pair of drakes dropped into the chop. The Chessie took her line on the far duck, bobbing belly up and soon the pair was lying beside the blind. The curly coat of the retriever showered her partners in recognition of their shooting and also just to let them know that just because the bay water was not frozen, doesn't mean it's not cold.

This scene was repeated throughout the morning, as whistlers, butterballs, and broadbills coursed back and forth nervously. The cork decoys, because of their size and weight rode through the wind and waves with incredible lifelike stability, luring many of the flocks within range.

The air around had intermittently showered them, but again it was difficult to tell exactly where the water came from; the heavens, the shore's pounding mist or the sly and loveable damp Chessie. The wind continued from the north, at times stronger than others, but always blowing, blowing, blowing. With reddened faces and fingers, they blazed away until they approached a legal limit.

For some mysterious reason there suddenly came the first lull in the morning's flights. It was then that the chill set in. They hadn't realized the temperature had dropped 25 degrees and the wind now blustered at times to 40 mph. It was not only the numbness of the fingers and toes, but a deep, damp, aching chill. They finally knew that it was mandatory they warm up a bit and dragged out their thermos' of hot coffee, tea and soup, which washed down sandwiches and large chunks of pound cake. Slowly, the inner ache subsided, even though their hands and feet were still frosty. They had no idea they were so cold, for their intensity in search of game and the adrenalin rush that accompanied the flocks of ducks had masked the fact, but this phenomenon had peaked awhile ago and from then on it was a slow cool slide.

They knocked down their final whistler and sat looking at one another, shivering and shaking, hoping the dog would volunteer to retrieve the decoys. The wind rushed through the rocks and the temperature plummeted further and as the snow blew horizontally, trying to reach the ground. A new look appeared on their faces. It was a look of fear, fear that whatever blew now from that black midday sky could end their duck hunting permanently. With cracking of their canvas coats, teeth chattering like nervous beavers, but now with purpose, they waded out to pick up as quickly as possible. One serious half-hour later, they climbed over the gunwales, started the outboard, and headed slowly home into the frigid wind. The heat generated by picking the blocks was gone in five minutes and as the spray broke over the bow, even the decoys appeared frozen stiff. They hit the dock a half an hour later with that bone chilling paralysis that made it an effort to climb out and pull the boat up onto its trailer.

The local establishment was two miles away and seemed a hundred at this point. To add insult to injury, the truck's heater blew cold and the windshield was intermittently coated with ice the entire distance. They pulled up short behind the restaurant and all three scrambled into the back room and stood there shivering. The owner, their friend and fellow duck hunter, could not begin to understand their slurred story but did comprehend immediately their plight and led them to the wood stove and hurriedly brought them a couple of large mugs of steaming hot coffee.

It took at least 45 to 50 minutes for the shivering, shaking and stammering to subside and it wasn't until then that the gravity of their situation sunk home. They had no idea they had been so cold, and they sat for hours drying out their clothes, inhaling food and drink, and reliving what went wrong and how to prevent it the next time. They thought they had been prepared and yet, still, came seriously close to severe hypothermia.

Like a self-contained and finely regulated furnace, the body maintains its core temperature under normal circumstances at 98.6, give or take a degree. When subjected to a cold environment, the body responds in essentially two ways. It increases heat production by rapid, rhythmic muscle contraction, or shivering. Shivering usually starts when the body's core temperature drops one or two degrees. The second mechanism whereby the body attempts to maintain its temperature is by shunting of blood away from the extremities, which have a large surface area and therefore high external heat loss and direct it more towards the trunk of the body, including the vital organs. This vascular shunting away from the hands and feet, and arms and legs, accounts for the poor circulation and inability to keep your toes and fingers warm without proper insulative covers. It also accounts for the mechanism and ease with which frostbite can occur.

Frostbite refers to a freezing of the appendages; digits of the hands and feet, and ears. Like burns, there are different degrees of freezing, those more superficial involving just the skin and resulting in temporarily swollen, reddened, and hypersensitive digits; all the way to deep, third degree or severe frostbite where the digits actually freeze completely and die permanently. Frostbite occurs more commonly than hypothermia and does so very subtly because of the anesthetic effect of cold. The appearance of frosty, white and insensitive skin signals early freezing. A sign of progressive frostbite is a rather sudden relief of pain, due to the frozen nerves inability to transmit this sensation. To prevent frostbite, all appendages of the body including the ears and nose should be protected from wind, water, and excessive cold. Rewarming and thus thawing frostbitten appendages should be done rather slowly. Ideally they are submerged in a warm water bath at 105 to 110 degrees. Be cautious getting too close to heaters or fires until the protective skin sensation returns. Rubbing the limb should be avoided for it can create abrasions and sloughing of the fragile insensate skin. Failure of sensory recovery or persistent darkness of the digits are clear indications to see a doctor.

In contrast to frostbite, hypothermia involves a cooling of the actual body's core. Technically, it develops when the body's temperature drops below 95 degrees Fahrenheit. Once cold has overwhelmed the body's defense mechanism, hypothermia can be rapidly progressive. The signs of hypothermia are subtle and may be appreciated only by knowledgeable individuals. Speech begins to slur when the body's core temperature drops two degrees below normal and muscle weakness develops with a three degree body temperature drop. If cold continues to dominate the body further, it rapidly overcomes the body's regulatory thermostat and all body processes slow down, which ultimately could lead to death. It is not a painful process but rather a sneaky, progressive paralysis, so early warning signals must be recognized and heeded.

When should one look at the thermometer and just stay home? Most winter sporting events held in North America will cancel when the mercury dips below -10 degrees F. Although humans have exercised at all temperatures without injury, this seems to be a prudent point to throw another log on the fire and pick up your favorite Gene Hill book until it warms up a bit.

Hypothermia can occur at temperatures above freezing for it is ultimately a result of the combination of temperature, wind velocity, duration of exposure and rate of temperature drop. We have all heard tell of the disaster that fell one bright and mild Armistice Day along the upper Mississippi bottoms in the late 1940's. The temperature dropped some 50 to 60 degrees within a few hours and many hunters were not able to acclimate either mentally or physically to that rate of change and perished.

Other predisposing factors that hunters should be aware of are fatigue, poor nutrition, or lengthy hunger, and the use of alcohol. It is more than mere myth that alcohol has a warming effect on the body. It is dangerous. As the body cools it shunts the blood away from the extremities to maintain its temperature. Alcohol works adversely by increasing blood flow to the extremities, thereby increasing heat loss and so we have another reason why alcohol should not be used before or during a hunt. For hunters with asthma or coronary artery disease, it's worth remembering that cold does increase the risk of attacks when exposed to extreme conditions.

The concept of heat transference is one always to keep in mind. This basically relates to heat being transferred away from the body more rapidly than it should be. One obvious way to prevent heat transference is to wear heavily insulated clothes. The use of air trapping materials, either natural such as wool or down, or synthetic such as dacron or thermax limits the flow of heat away from the body. The effect of these air trapping fabrics however can be negated if they become damp, or if the wind is strong. Therefore, it is mandatory to wear some type of wind breaking material with a close knit weave.

Dampness likewise speeds the transference of heat away from the body. This can be demonstrated in no more dramatic fashion than an individual totally submersed in icy water and how their life sustaining heat can be drawn away from them, even to death within ten to fifteen minutes. Some of the synthetics such as thermax, polypropylene and dacron, as well as wool, can provide insulation even when wet, however are not nearly as effective as when dry. It is of upmost importance to stay dry. Gortex fabric has drastically improved this possibility and is well worth the extra cost. Vinyl and rubberized fabrics don't allow for perspiration release and after a few hours the hunter may find himself wet from within. The results are the same, increased heat loss.

Layering clothes has long been practiced by hunters as well as other athletes, particularly skiers and cold weather runners. Exercising the body, even in cold weather, causes perspiration and depending on the level of activity, this perspiration can dampen some or all of the clothes worn. With this in mind, if one anticipates a bout of physical activity such as setting decoys or walking briskly to a hilltop deer blind, layer down to an acceptable level and then once the physical exertion has ceased, allow the body to cool down, the air to evaporate as much perspiration as possible, and then pull out and slip on your outer insulating layer of clothes for the still hunt.

One final aspect of heat transference when the hunt involves a lengthy sit, is the seat itself. Sitting on insulative type materials such as a five gallon plastic bucket, wooden seat, driftwood logs, or one of the commercially available insulite seating pads are much more desireable and effective than sitting for a long while on cold stones, frozen stumps, or any metal structures. Twenty-five to thirty percent of all body heat is lost from the head and scalp. Therefore, waterproof, insulative head gear can never be underestimated.

Cold injuries are to be taken seriously by all who hunt in less temperate climates. If early hypothermia is suspected, a brief, but brisk walk or other form of physical activity will help increase body metabolism. The body can also gain heat from external objects such as fires, the sun, or warm foods and fluids. The preparation and prevention are paramount, but early recognition of cold injuries usually will prevent disasters.

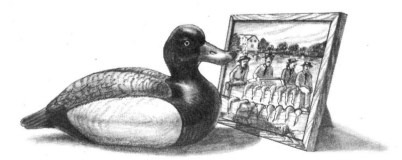

Appendix

For your convenience this quick reference section, containing the exercises explained in this book, has been developed. Please use this guide to develop an exercise program that best fits your needs. The Weekly Training Schedule below will help you plan your week.

In each exercise box there is a number (i.e. 4-1). The first number refers to the chapter and the second number, the order in which it appears within the chapter (i.e. 4-1 appears in chapter 4 as the 1st figure). Please refer to the chapter exercises for further explanation and rationale of each exercise.

Weekly Training Schedule

Monday	Tuesday	Wednesday	Thursday	Friday	Saturday	Sunday
Flexibility Training—10 min. Low impact Aerobics—30-45 min.	Flexibility Training—10 min. Weight Training—60 min.	Rest or Light Walk	Flexibility Training—10 min. Low impact Aerobics—30-45 min.	Flexibility Training—10 min. Weight Training—60 min.	Rest or Light Walk	Flexibility Training—10 min. Hunt Specific Training—1-3 hrs.

Measuring Your Ideal Cardiac Capacity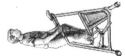

220 - your age x 80% = Aerobic Heart Rate

TABLE 1: *Specific Exercises—Trunk*

NECK

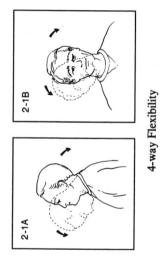

2-1A   2-1B

4-way Flexibility

BACK

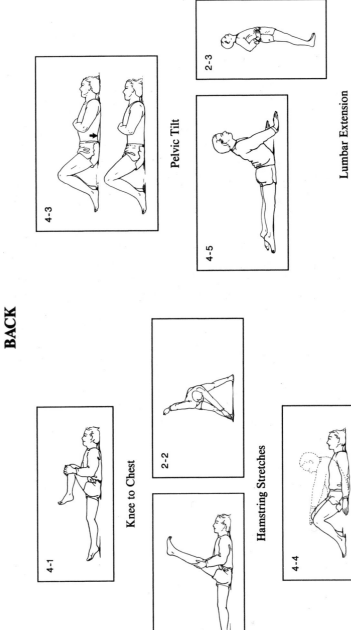

4-3

Pelvic Tilt

2-3

4-5

Lumbar Extension

4-1

Knee to Chest

2-2

4-2

Hamstring Stretches

4-4

Partial Sit-up = Crunches

TABLE 2: *Specific Exercises—Upper Extremity*

SHOULDER

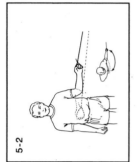

5-1

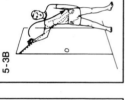

5-2

Free Weights—Side Lifts = Fly

Rotation—Internal and External

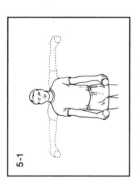

5-3A

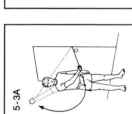

5-3B

Functional Exercise = Create Your Own

ELBOW/FOREARM

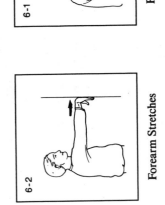

6-2

Forearm Stretches

6-1

Free Weight Wrist Curls

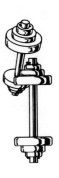

Appendix continues on next page.

TABLE 3: Specific Exercises—Lower Extremity

HIP/KNEE

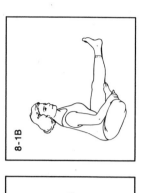

2-4

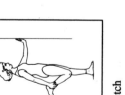

8-1A

Quadricep Stretch

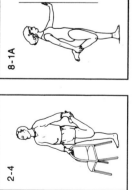

2-5

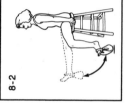

8-1B

Hamstring Stretch

2-7

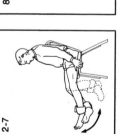

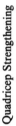

8-2

Quadricep Strengthening